CALORIES
in
CALORIES
out

CALORIES
in
CALORIES
out

What It Took for Me to Lose 140 Pounds—And How You Can Do It Too

AARON KNIPP

CONTENTS

Advice from the Fat Kid

At nineteen, I ate like a child: If it wasn't deep fried or wrapped in a tortilla, I did not want anything to do with it. Let me walk you through a day in the life of Aaron: I would start by eating an entire pizza on my own with a large soda to wash it down. Once that had settled, I'd be on the hunt for anything sweet—until my next meal, of course. Fast forward to 10:00 p.m. when my buddies and I would be on our routine Taco Bell run. I know what you're thinking: We all eat; it's not so crazy to indulge occasionally. This wasn't your average bad day. This was my every day. I was regularly consuming at least 5,000–6,000 calories a day. That's three full meals, seconds, thirds, and snacks. No nineteen-year-old—or anyone for that matter—should be consuming anywhere near that many calories. I did, all without any kind of exercise to offset my eating habits.

Being fat was just a part of me. It was like breathing, it came so naturally. As crazy as it is to think about now, that lifestyle felt completely normal. It's the only life I'd known since day one. I started as a chunky baby and only seemed to get bigger from there. Growing up overweight is a completely different experience than gaining weight later in life as an adult. If you've grown up within five to ten pounds of a healthy weight but then gain excess pounds later, you know why it's so disheartening to be fat. You have lived the difference. But when you're that big from the start, you don't know any other kind of life. Nothing specific caused my weight gain: I had loving parents, friends, and there was no trauma or stress that brought me to that point. I was just a fat kid, period.

Now brace yourself, because this Former Fat Kid is about to say what every person who has ever tried to motivate you to lose weight has already said. You ready?

Your quality of life will be infinitely better once you lose the weight.

Infinitely better.

If you're already rolling your eyes at me, I totally understand. This is the point at which the old Aaron would throw this book out the window. "Your quality of life will be better" is the most annoying phrase to hear from a fit person. It's easy for them to say. They're not big, so they don't know what it's like. I'm stubborn, and hearing people tell me that just made me want to prove them wrong. Here's the issue: 99 out of 100 times, the people telling you this have absolutely no idea what they're saying or what they're asking you to do. They watched a video where someone talked about the quality of life, and they're trying to be helpful. They latched onto a motivational saying, and they want to pass it on. *But they don't know what they're saying because they haven't been where you are.*

I've seen both sides.

Long story short, I used to be obese—like can't-touch-my-toes-if-I-tried kind of big. At nineteen years old, I stood over six feet tall and weighed **320 pounds**. In a moment of realization, I picked up my phone and started scouring the web for tips on how to lose 100 pounds. It took me almost two years, but I did it. I lost 140 pounds! I made a ton of mistakes along the way, but I learned from them, kept on pushing, and I made it to the other side.

How did I do it? It wasn't like I hadn't tried to lose weight before. I'd tried everything. I'd done it all: read books, tried the diets, and suffered through you-need-to-be-healthier lectures from my parents, doctors, and even my friends. None of it worked for me. If you're even remotely close to how overweight I was, then my guess is that none of those methods—diets, plans, or guilt-trips—have worked or will work for you either.

Simply put, I figured it out on my own. I sifted through a bunch of crap out there on weight loss (and believe me—people have opinions, and not all of them are good ones), and I found a rhythm that worked for me. This is the book I needed when I was losing weight—the book I wished someone would have given me when I felt hopeless. I want to save you from the bullshit, and walk you through, plain and simple, what I did to lose 140 pounds.

If you want to lose weight, and you're looking for a sign—this is it. This book is your sign. Let's get started.

CHAPTER ONE

Weight Loss for Real Life

L ife is different for you when you're in shape: you feel better about yourself, and you notice how people start treating you better because of it. It was something I was not used to. The old me would have never been comfortable going into a nutrition shop. It's a whole different world in there. The employees are all fit, the men are massive, the women are strong; it's a place for healthy, fit people to thrive. The kind of place where an overweight person like me walked in and thought, "Damn, I wish I looked like that."

What's crazy is, now that I'm fit, something as simple as a trip to get a smoothie feels like a whole new experience. What seemed like a scary place to me once is now my happy place. I love going there. I've made it to a place in my weight loss where I feel confident around all these fitness buffs and can actually relate to them.

The other day I took my buddy into my favorite nutrition shop and had one of those out-of-body experiences. My friend is a great person. He's no body builder and not fat by any means. He's a slender guy who fits the average mold of what "born skinny" looks like. I brought him here before our work-out and assumed he'd be accepted. But that didn't seem to be the case. I watched how the cashier politely smiled at him but didn't pay him too much attention. Odd to me—since she's the same person I talk to daily. She greeted me warmly and asked how I liked the pre-workout she had recommended me a few days prior.

I watched as my friend walked around just looking at what they had to offer; he wasn't really interested in anything and didn't seem like this was a place for him. I found it so strange, but it reminded me of my first time in this very shop. At that time, I didn't look anything like I do now. I was 300 pounds and had come in with a friend who frequented the place. I was just getting into the fitness side of my journey and didn't feel like I should be in a place like this. I remember how the cashier that day greeted my friend, asked him questions about his workouts, brought him a sample of a new supplement that had just arrived. While I stood there feeling invisible, I couldn't help but feel like an outsider. Smoothies, supplements, and pre-workouts all sounded foreign to me. I kept my head down that day feeling the pangs of the fat, ignored friend. Fast forward to today, and I never thought of what it would be like to be on the other end of the spectrum, to be the regular those employees greeted and were excited to see. I realized then what makes the difference is your drive, your commitment to this lifestyle. Now my head is held high when I walk in three to four times a week; it's me who gets offered cool new products and the occasional free shake. I had to take a moment to appreciate how much has changed. It's not until I was living it that I stopped to think, "I *do* belong here."

The Transformation

Today, I look and feel like a completely different person than nineteen-year-old Aaron. People who haven't seen me since my transformation hardly recognize me. I have bulked up to 200 pounds and slimmed down my body fat percentage. I pushed myself to go to the gym, and now I actually enjoy it. I go because I want to keep improving myself. My relationship with weight loss has been a complete 180-degree turnaround. Instead of being the token fat friend, I'm the fit one in my friend group to whom they come for advice. People who see me at the gym ask about my routines and how to do certain exercises. That boy munching on fast food would have never thought this day would come.

Like I said, I was nineteen years old when I actually started to make progress on my weight loss journey. This wasn't my first time attempting to lose weight—not even close to it. One aspect of my life that has been constant, thanks to growing up big, is the various get-skinny-quick diets and training programs I've tried since I was a kid. My parents hired personal trainers for me—not when I was a child, of course, but when I started getting a little older around middle school and throughout high school. I tried every option available to me. I followed weight loss shows, read books, and even listened to inspirational speakers. I bought protein shakes, nutrition bars, and every supplement in the book. You name it, I tried it.

Let's do some math: say that I tried, in a concerted effort, to lose weight three times a year, starting at age thirteen. That would mean that, at the moment of my turning point, I had tried to lose weight—and **failed**—eighteen times. And that's a conservative estimate. That's eighteen excruciating times I tried to lose weight and was only left feeling defeated.

at the moment of my turning point, I had tried to lose weight—and failed— eighteen times

In retrospect, I can see that there were two main problems with the programs, plans, and workouts I tried before. First and foremost, those plans were not made for real life. With so many plans, they ask you to buy meal plans, protein bars, meal supplements, or shakes. Each company has you buying specific meals from them in order to see results—you just can't do that forever. I know I wasn't able to do it. I was nineteen and in college; do you think I wanted to spend all my time and the little money on these companies that "promised" results? No! I wanted to be a normal college kid who went out with his friends. A few years later I turned twenty-one, and no twenty-one-year-old in their right mind is going to bring their Atkins bar to the club—they're just not going to! It doesn't matter how dedicated you are; it's not going to happen. I can promise you there is no alcoholic drink allowed in any of those diets, and for a lot of people, it's pretty unrealistic to think that they're never, ever going to drink.

These plans are great for short periods of time. They can help you lose ten to twenty pounds. If you want a genuine lifestyle change, the majority of widely marketed, publicized plans are not going to work. No matter how committed you want to be, it's not going to a sustainable diet, and you will find yourself back at square one.

The second thing is what I call "a reason why." You have to know why you're trying to lose weight to stay committed. You can't run on pure motivation alone. You can't just lean on adrenaline. Let's say you're super motivated to lose weight for an upcoming event; you'll probably stay motivated for a few weeks—and that's wonderful! Congratulations! I'm very happy you found something to aim for. But that motivation will fade when the event arrives. It's understandable; you're only human! When that motivation is gone, what are you left with? What is something you can reasonably achieve? You've got to have a reason to keep losing weight! I can't stress this enough. A lifestyle change is not a get-skinny-quick scheme, so find YOUR reason!

The plans and diets I tried before (eighteen plus times) didn't provide a good reason for me to lose weight, and they didn't provide sustainability. It's the same story with weight loss shows. It didn't matter how many different weight loss shows I watched; I never felt that I could relate to the contestants. Their lives were nothing like mine; their lives were simulations. They didn't face normal pressures or social situations that someone my age experienced. They had the world watching them and intense regimens, and, yes, the people on those shows lose weight. Of course they do, but I was not living in fit camp: I was in college, living in a dorm. I couldn't imitate the simulated situations on the shows. I needed something that fit my needs for my weight goals to be achieved.

One hundred and forty pounds later, I'm here to provide something different. I'm going to lay it all out for you. It's actually very simple. I'm a point A to point B kind of guy. My friends and family (everyone who suggested all those other plans in the first place) can attest that I always look for the path of least resistance. I'm here to make this process simple for you and to break down weight loss to its most basic elements. I'm going to cut the crap, cut the confusion, and just lead you through my process.

You've got to have a reason to keep losing weight!

I can't promise you the perfect plan to optimal physical health. I'll tell you up front that I never gave up fast food and my diet is definitely not what a nutritionist would set out as an ideal model. I'm not here to tell you how to achieve an optimal BMI, how to gain muscle, or how to turn the extra flab around your waist into a six pack. I will not give you a stack of charts or make you a health expert. I'm a practical guy, and I am as busy and tired as the next person, so when I went through this process, I could really only focus on one goal: losing weight. I'm not here promising perfection, but I can attest that these methods are effective.

What I really want you to understand is that there's hope. It was a very long and tough road, but if I could figure it out on my own, then I know you can do it, too. Milestone by milestone, I hit my goals and kept pressing on. Being under 300 pounds for the first time was, of course, a big deal to me. Hitting 249 made a big impression: that was the first time in five to six years that I was closer to 200 pounds than 300. More than either of these, though, the 220-mark felt significant to me. It's when I—a six-foot-one-inch male—went from fat to chubby. I had already gone from obese to fat, but 220 was when I felt I had crossed over into "normal" territory. I was certainly on the high end of normal, but I was in a thicker part of the pre-existing bell curve. I remember thinking, "I can shop most places now." Being 220 pounds was the first time I felt normal. Granted, I still needed to lose another forty pounds, but it was an important mark for me. I knew that some of my friends weighed 205 pounds, and I felt that 220 and 205 weren't that far apart.

What I really want you to understand is that there's hope

When I got down to 200, for the first time in my life I had friends who weighed more than me. I thought it was crazy that I could "weigh less" than someone. Growing up, I was always the heaviest one in the group. Always. Never was there a person in my age group that I met who weighed more than I did. Reaching a point where I was able to be compared to the others around AND even weigh less than someone was a huge and new world for me.

Small, everyday experiences have become pleasant reminders of how far I've come. When I'm at a buddy's house and forget a shirt for after a swim, I can just borrow one. That may seem like nothing to some, but for a long time that wasn't a possibility for me. If my friends wanted to go from the pool to get something to eat, and I didn't bring extra clothes, I was out of luck. I couldn't borrow anyone else's clothes. They wouldn't fit! Even in middle school, I had trouble finding clothes to borrow. I'd spend weeks at my best friend's home in the summer, and if I forgot something, his mom would bring out her husband's clothes—not my friend's. His dad, of course, was an adult and much larger than a child. Here I was in seventh grade wearing a grown man's clothes and even they were tight on me.

A recent visit to one of my favorite Mexican restaurants reminded me of just how much I've accomplished. It was one of my family's favorite places to go when I was growing up. We'd go there for birthdays or just a weekend night out, and it has a special place in my heart. No one makes a cheese crisp like they can . . . trust me, I've looked! I've been there count-less times in my life; one particular time though, is seared into my memory because it's when I noticed I needed to change.

Since moving into my dorm at GCU, I hadn't had the chance to go in for one of those iconic cheese crisps, so when a few friends wanted to go, I was super excited! There were four of us going, so we wanted to sit in a booth. When we went to sit down, I literally could not fit in the seat. The chairs were bolted into the floor to keep from moving when people got in, and nothing was budging. I was trapped. In all the times I had been to this restaurant, I had never had this problem. I didn't want to make a big deal of it, so I sucked in my gut and squeezed myself into the booth. It was so uncomfortable. I had to force myself in, but I didn't fit. No matter how I maneuvered my body, the table was still digging into my stomach. I remember feeling so embarrassed while also in physical pain. None of my friends said anything, but it's obvious when someone doesn't fit in a booth. Their expressions were clear to read: *Poor guy, how embarrassing.*

I can still tell you in which booth I was stuck. It's a surreal experience to sit there now and see how much space I have. I sit in the booth and, I swear, you could fit a whole ruler between my stomach and the table. Two people could sit on my lap and still have plenty of room. I could have my legs criss-cross on the booth and still have space. It's insane to imagine how big I once was when I see where I am now. Marker by marker, pound by pound, I was able to reach my goal.

You Need a Plan

If I could go back and tell 320-pound Aaron anything, I would give him this book. I looked for a guide, for someone to show me what to do, and I just didn't have anyone. There was nothing out there that worked for me.

The biggest struggle in the world was learning how to lose weight. I wasted so much time and energy during the first part of my weight loss journey because I had no idea what I was doing. The first year I lost fifty pounds and I struggled.

I want you to enjoy as much of your life as possible

If I could condense it, I would. Realistically, if you're 320 pounds and you are trying to get down to 180, the first fifty pounds should fall off easily. You'll see it on any Hulu and Netflix shows—it happens in roughly three weeks. But you have to have someone tell you what to do. If someone could have just told me what foods to eat and what exercises to do, it would have been a faster, more productive process.

The one thing I had was determination. I had more drive than I'd ever had in my life. I would have dropped out of college to make this happen if I needed to. That didn't seem to be enough, though. I was running on all cylinders, wasting time, making mistakes, and I didn't know what I was doing.

But I didn't need to exhaust myself: all I was missing was a concentrated plan tailored to me.

The second year, I finally hit my stride, figured out my process, and just like that lost another ninety pounds. The whole process still took two years, and I was absolutely miserable the whole time. I did not get to enjoy the ages of nineteen and twenty because I spent so much time trying to figure out a routine.

If I had been given the tools and guidance necessary, imagine the possibilities.

How cool would it have been if I knew what to do from the start? What if I had lost the weight in six months or one year? How different would it have been for me to be in college and to be in shape?

I want to save you the time and effort I wasted. I want you to enjoy as much of your life as possible. The first step to change is realizing that you're not where you want to be. I'm going to start my story with where I began: although I didn't realize it at the time, allowing myself to stay content as "the fat boy" really sucked.

CHAPTER TWO

Shitty Normal

Being overweight has its challenges. I was always tired, always hungry, and never felt like there was a place for my body type. The worst part? That was normal to me— shitty normal, but I didn't know any other life. Whether you're twenty pounds or 220 pounds overweight the world we live in makes you feel like you are different. You have a different perception of life than someone who is fit. It's difficult to even realize your view is so warped until you do finally get in shape.

> *The reality is that you are already living in a hell of your own creation; the only difference is you've convinced yourself that it's normal*

At 320 pounds, I told myself I was fine, but I was far from healthy. So if you hear that little voice in your head say that you're okay, know that you may be at a functional level, but you're not where you could be. The reality is that you are already living in a hell of your own creation; the only difference is you've convinced yourself that it's normal.

Before we dive into the routines of losing weight, it is essential that you fully understand the reason you've decided to change. If you do not understand the depth of what it is costing you—physically and emotionally—to stay overweight, you will be tempted to give up during the process. Believe me: It is so incredibly easy to seize any opportunity to avoid doing the work I'm challenging you to do. It's a tough process, and if you don't know to your core why you are putting yourself through hell to reach your goal, then you will go back to what you know.

Physical Weight

There are two categories which keep you down as an obese person—two big ways in which your quality of life is low. There are the physical problems you face and also the emotional problems. I'll start with the physical.

Sweat. When it comes to the physical discomfort of being overweight, I instantly think of sweat. Perhaps it's the inner fat kid in me, but I absolutely hate sweating. I have a visceral reaction to the thought of it. I even hate the word sweat. It's unpleasant to hear and even grosser to see. It brings me back to a very uncomfortable time.

When I was big, I would sweat all the time. It wasn't the kind of sweat a quick change of a T-shirt could fix. When I say I would sweat, I mean constantly—not just when it was hot, not just when I was walking around, and not just when

I was sitting on a leather seat. It didn't matter what the hell I did or what I didn't do or what the weather was, I was sweaty.

If I got up from the couch, my back was sweaty.

Going from one class to another just down the hall, drenched.

Driving in my car, soaked in sweat.

Laying in my bed at night, you guessed it . . . sweating.

Every second of every day I was made to feel uncomfortable, thanks to my body's constant perspiration.

Every second of every day was covered in sweat.

It was so damn gross, terribly uncomfortable, and straight up embarrassing. I couldn't help but feel ashamed. Nobody wants to be around someone emanating BO, and there was no hiding it with me. The most ridiculous part of it all was that I ignored my sweat's connection to my weight. Sweating made up so much of my existence that I eventually just accepted that my body temperature was just, naturally and unfortunately, higher than other people's.

I ignored my sweat's connection to my weight

It's laughable now because, in hindsight, it is clear to me that I was ignorant to my own body trying to tell me there was something wrong. I would be doing nothing, just sitting down in class or in a restaurant and I. Was. Sweating. That kind of sweat is not normal, and I was all too willing to ignore that sign.

I remember in high school and middle school, walking from the car to class or even to the second story of a building would put me out of breath. Something as simple as walking across campus, an activity other people didn't think twice about, would exhaust me. I didn't question that experience or think, "Other people don't feel this way after walking up stairs." I just accepted it. And I know a ton of other people who are the same way—and they just accept it as well. I couldn't imagine that there was a possible reality for me where I wasn't sweating all the time. I've learned now that there is! I had to work for it (read the rest of the book to see how), but that sweat-free life was available to me. I didn't have to feel gross moving from the car to my front door. I didn't have to run out of breath going up the stairs.

If this resonates with you, know that I understand feeling resistant to blaming sweat on your weight. I know how difficult it is to accept that being overweight influences daily life in such a shitty way. I wish I could blame it on genetics, and you might be tempted to do that as well, but you can't. You might have bad genetics; I have bad genetics, but genetics is more of a hindrance than a condition. Just because you are short doesn't mean you will never reach the high cupboards. You just need a stepstool. Genetics are out of our control. We do not get to pick and choose what our parents give us. We can, however, control how we treat our bodies and what we put in them. Lose the weight, and you won't have to deal with pools of sweat all the time.

Next, I need to address clothing. Like most kids, I cared about what I wore. I wanted to fit in and wear the cool clothes I saw other people wearing. Feeling good about what you're wearing gives you confidence. When you dress like shit, you feel like shit, and other people can tell. Here's the problem though: nothing existed in my size. I understand that not everyone cares about fashion. But when you're obese, your style options are limited, and you don't get to add that unique flair of your own style. You are lucky if you can find anything in your size at all. I don't mean just the stylish clothes; I mean normal, everyday clothes. Most places don't have a big and tall section. You can completely rule out any normal, name-brand place. I can remember walking into a clothing store at the mall and recognizing a look of surprise on the faces of the employees. They'd say, "Can we help you?" but the terror in their faces told me that they didn't have anything in their store for me.

The worst part was when, miraculously, I did find something—a shirt or a pair of pants I liked—the pieces never seemed to work for me. Even when I bought something I liked, something that even technically fit, I still never felt good about it. I never looked at myself in the dressing room and said, "Yes! This looks really good on me!" Everything I wore looked like a variation of the last shirt; it offered no personality, no style, and I was just thankful it fit. My clothes were baggy, neutral, and just plain boring. I couldn't find attractive clothes, and when I found something that fit, it cost me extra money for being a plus size. That's three extra dollars for a shirt that doesn't even look good. It was a lose-lose situation.

The fact is, when you aren't able to find clothes that fit you, you start to resent yourself and lose any kind of interest in taking care of yourself. This attitude makes it more and more difficult to find motivation to dress yourself and take care of your body. It's a cycle which reinforces itself. When you can look in the mirror and like your reflection, you start to care about the person you see.

Lastly, I want to talk about energy. Energy is one of those topics which, because of my history, still irritates me. Even typing the word makes every part of the inner fat kid in me cringe. Doctors and trainers lecture overweight people on energy. It always pissed me off because, clearly, these people had never been in my shoes. They had no right to tell me how I felt during the day. Their warnings about low-energy levels felt hollow to me—just something to say to the fat kid.

Everything I wore looked like a variation of the last shirt; it offered no personality, no style, and I was just thankful it fit

Having lived through that transformation, though, I can now tell you firsthand that your energy levels do change. Looking back on my old routines, I have no idea how I functioned in my everyday life. My productivity was extremely low. I was tired all the time, and I never wanted to do anything.

This is what a routine day off (no school or work) would look like for me:

10:00 a.m.–1:00 p.m. - Slow wake up

1:00–5:00 p.m. - A meal and whatever errands I needed to do that day

5:00–9:00 p.m. - Going out for a casual meal and relaxing on the couch

9:00–10:00 p.m. - Another late-night meal

10:00–11:00 p.m. - Transition to bed

Even if I stretched this schedule out to fit in another hour of productivity, it allows, at best, five hours to get some-thing—anything—done. I wouldn't have stayed as fat as I did if I had cho-sen another activity besides resting. My rest was sustaining my obesity, and I felt tired every minute. That's just what naturally happens when you're that big. I didn't necessarily need to take a nap after four or five hours of doing things, but I definitely felt like I needed to be at home and relax. I would lie around on the couch for a few hours before I let myself go to bed.

My productivity was extremely low. I was tired all the time, and I never wanted to do anything

Taking a look at the big picture though, it's easy to see that I hardly had any time left for work or even for outside projects. Think of all the activities I was missing out on, simply because I was carrying around extra weight! My inactivity was not a sustainable way of life.

How much I was sweating, what I could wear, and how much energy I had were all daily physical limitations as an obese person. As one might expect, I did not participate in sports—neither as a child nor as an adult. I just couldn't keep up; it meant dealing with aches and pains in my bones and muscles that they were not used to. A healthy person might ache after sitting in one place for too long or after sleeping with an uncomfortable pillow. Add 100-plus pounds to that experience, and that was my situation: constantly in pain from the pressure and strain of carrying around extra weight. I'm not a doctor, but I know that aches and pains are just the tip of the iceberg as far as risks related to obesity. Ask your physician, and I'm sure they'll be able to give you a long list. But I'm not here to tell you what everyone else tells you. Chances are, if you've been to the doctor in the last six months, they've already given you a lecture. What I'm trying to show you is my life at my largest weight was no way for someone so young to live. More than I knew at the time, more than I was able to put into words, the pounds on my body made me feel like garbage.

the pounds on my body made me feel like garbage

There is nothing you could give me now to go back to that life. Absolutely nothing. The physical problems, however, weren't even the worst of it.

Emotional Weight

When it comes to the social and emotional aspects of being overweight, I'm a realist. It's not fun to talk about, but it's actually a huge part of the everyday hell of a fat person. When you are overweight, you're not only carrying around extra physical pounds, you are also carrying around the weight of other people's judgment and opinions. Just like the physical weight has physical ramifications, the emotional weight has emotional ramifications.

I'll get right to it: being comfortable in your own skin is harder when you're obese. When you're not comfortable with your own body, you put out that energy making others feel you are unapproachable. I remember how self-conscious I would feel doing anything; it always feels as if people are projecting their ideas of what you should weigh onto you. That builds a wall between you and the world. Society has its idea of what healthy people should look like and eat, which creates a stigma that if you're overweight you don't care about yourself. I try to remember that people aren't doing this maliciously. It happens subconsciously because it was what we were all taught: "Fat is bad. Fat is unhealthy. Fat isn't pretty." The sad truth is that, even when people don't mean to, they judge you.

being comfortable in your own skin is harder when you're obese

As anyone overweight knows, there are telltale signs that just being yourself is making someone else feel uneasy. It's never obvious, it's something you grow accustomed to seeing: the shifting of eyes when you're getting a coffee, or people staring at your order. It could be a cold shoulder, or even someone just pretending you don't exist. This isn't just something obese people deal with—the world treats people badly no matter their size. That's just the reality of it, but when these cues become constant you know what's causing it. It's almost as if you've got the flu and people are avoiding you. Except you don't. So why are people so quick to keep their distance?

One thing you must remember is that you can't control people's reactions or judgments. Not everyone is rude, and there are those who don't judge you for what's on the outside but who you are on the inside. We can't put everyone in the world in the same category, otherwise we are no better. My experience showed me that the majority of people are uneasy around anyone who doesn't fit the "normal" standard; those who seem abnormal in any sense get treated differently. Abnormal is a harsh word, one I try not to use lightly. I use it for two reasons, the first being that's how I felt when people stared or judged me; the second is because 140 extra pounds does make a difference on the human body. Irregular is perhaps a more polite term. Either way, any person walking down the street with that many extra pounds is bound to cause a few double takes. Statistically, 320 pounds on a nineteen-year-old is an irregular size.

If you are overweight, you understand exactly what I'm talking about. You know the social cues and your heart drops when you see them. There were times when I'd ordered food and, no matter if healthy or not, I would catch the raise of the brow from the cashier. Almost mocking me, making me worry if I had ordered too much or not enough of the healthy options that showed I was trying to change. It's a very uncomfortable feeling, wondering if your order is the appropriate amount of food—in the other person's estimation. I don't know if many people have ever had this thought.

Perhaps the reason people find the extra weight so off-putting is the stereotypes that come with being overweight: that we are lazy and don't care about ourselves. In my experience (let's remember I've been on both sides of this equation), people are less likely to relate to your problems or show sympathy to anything you've experienced when you're above a certain weight. They'll look at you as if you did this to yourself, and it's your problem, not theirs.

The impact of people's casual criticism eventually starts to take a toll on you. You start believing that their opinions and judgments are a direct reflection of who you are. Instead of having pride in yourself, you feel ashamed and hide yourself. The downward cycle starts there: the moment we allow negative thoughts to stop us from living a full life. You create a warped reality where you are in constant paranoia that others are judging you because you've begun to judge yourself instead of helping yourself.

I think if those of us who are overweight only had to deal with the occasional jackass, we'd be fine. Just like everyone else, we'd bounce back because it wouldn't be our everyday. It wouldn't affect us that much. You have to understand though: This kind of shit happens every day! On top of what I've already mentioned, there are plenty of little events which add up to make it clear that others feel uncomfortable with your weight. In a million little ways, the world will try to tell you that you are not good enough, that you are worthless, and that people hate you. All of which are untrue. You are worth it, and you are capable.

The physical limitations of weight are already enough of a trial. To have to deal with other people's judgment—on top of those other challenges—just feels so unfair. Having that constant feeling that people around you are making assumptions about you messes with your head and leaves you with a feeling that stays long after the weight is gone. I can remember hanging out with my friends at Chipotle, having a nagging feeling in the pit of my stomach that they were all annoyed that I was there. I thought to myself, "I'm not thin enough to be around these people." These were my friends! I had no evidence to believe that they were judging me like that or annoyed at my presence. In fact, they invited me to come to lunch with them every time they went out. Regardless of the truth of the matter, though, I projected my feelings of worthlessness on them. Due to how many times I had experienced other people's stares and comments, I was worried, and part of me believed that even those close to me felt the same way. I grew paranoid.

The paranoia also played out with strangers. If I started chatting with someone, I'd immediately think, "This person is disgusted with even the idea of talking with me." I'd think this before people had a chance to respond or show that they were actually kind people. Looking back on that time in my life, I realize now that people probably judged me less often than I worried they did. But it didn't matter: All those times when I had been judged had already paved the way in my mind for more judgment. I saw dismay everywhere, and I experienced the feeling of being judged, even when it was all just in my head. It was a state of paranoia that consistently tore down my confidence.

These experiences operate in a vicious cycle. The criticism leads to paranoia, and paranoia erodes your confidence. When your self-esteem is low, you attract more negative energy, and the cycle begins again. If you don't like yourself, others will not like you, which in turn makes you hate yourself. It influences your confidence, how you take care of your own appearance, your feeling of self-worth, your energy, drive, and your overall happiness. It messes with your mental state and keeps you down longer.

Let's be honest: this right here—your life as it is—it's not the life you want forever

For me, self-confidence was always a struggle, I did not trust myself. I could not make decisions on my own, even if the decisions only influenced me. I wouldn't go to class without asking someone about my clothing choice. If I wanted to go grab food—even if I was going by myself—I'd text my buddies and see what sounded good to them. If they agreed that it was a good day for burritos, then I'd head to the burrito place. If they suggested Burger King, I'd go there. I was never the first to share my thoughts in a social setting; I kept to myself most of the time. I was scared to contradict anyone else or to have my own opinions. When my friends went to see a new movie, I'd ask their opinion before saying anything. I didn't even mean to do it; I had just convinced myself that I wasn't worthy of having my own opinions. You don't see just how much you're holding yourself back by not being confident in who you are.

People don't talk about the emotional aspect of being overweight, but it has a massive impact on your quality of life. Lack of confidence and paranoia follow you wherever you go. The constant thought that people are uncomfortable with you as a person can influence every aspect of your life: dating, making friends, and applying for jobs. Even something as simple as going to the grocery store can become a nightmare. The physical and emotional weight of being obese makes for a painful and exhausting existence, one in which a cycle of low confidence and paranoia pulls you down.

Although I didn't realize it, I was living under a lot of constant strain. And, if I'm even close to how you've felt, just know your life could be better. You excuse the damaging behavior because you don't know how great it could actually be. Let's be honest: this right here—your life as it is—it's not the life you want forever.

Now I'm going to share with you the moment that finally put me over the edge. It was the moment that I decided the cycle was going to end. This shit was not for me anymore.

CHAPTER THREE

My Turning Point

M y real journey began on December 11, 2012. All it took was one seemingly insignificant event, and my life turned around. It sounds crazy, but it's true: there is always a turning point. Something clicked for me, and I found an internal drive that I never had before. I decided to get in shape and, this time, I was able to follow through.

Girl at the Grill

I was a sophomore living on campus at Grand Canyon University. Remember, I weighed 320 pounds, which for a man my age and height was about 130-150 pounds overweight. Every night around nine o'clock, my group of friends and I found ourselves in the student commons. Here, students could buy food and drinks. There were several booths and tables for people to chill and hang out. It was a typical night for us. We were sitting adjacent to the grill where you could go for a late-night snack. My friends were done with class for the day and just wanted to relax. As they all chatted about their day, I was looking around the room, half listening to them but mostly people watching. I'd always felt it was the best place, other than Disneyland, to observe random people as they walked by.

That's when it happened: I saw this girl.

I know. I know this sounds cliché. Honestly, I've only told about five people this story because it sounds like the beginning of a rom com—and I can promise you I cringe at it—but I want to be honest with you. I wish I was making this story up, but this is exactly how it happened.

She was standing in line at the grill. I watched in awe because I had never seen a girl this beautiful before. I found her absolutely stunning, no exaggeration! I developed the most dramatic crush I've ever experienced in that moment. There was a fire inside of me when I watched her laugh, and I wanted to learn everything I could about her.

It's important to know that the old Aaron wasn't exactly a ladies' man. My self-worth and confidence had always been at an all-time low when it came to women. Not to mention my fear that, if I did get the courage to walk up to anyone, I'd be drenched in sweat before I even reached her. I put my head down. What was the point? I was sure that she wouldn't go for someone with my physique. I felt completely defeated and helpless—and I hadn't even spoken to her.

Of course, this wasn't my first encounter with an attractive woman. Sometimes I had the confidence to say something, while other times I let the moment pass. This time felt so much different than the rest. I remember sitting there and having an overwhelming sense of shame. I felt ashamed about the way I looked and the way I treated myself. How could I have let myself get to this point? I felt lonely and powerless, like the very definition of a mess. I thought, "You have absolutely no chance of ever dating this girl." My thoughts and feelings rushed through me, and this time they were hitting me hard.

I did the awkward move where you sneak sideways glances at a person—while trying to act casual (real smooth). A few minutes had passed; she picked up her food and, just like that, she was gone. I continued the rest of the night with my friends, without mentioning any of this to them.

Later, I went back to my dorm as usual, but that night I didn't sleep. I jumped on my computer and spent the whole night Googling how to lose weight. I read about the difference between fasting, eating "clean," and dieting. I studied how our bodies use food for energy and what exercise does to burn fat and keep us healthy. I can't say that one night of research made me an expert, but something had changed in me, and I was more motivated than I'd ever been.

something had changed in me, and I was more motivated than I'd ever been

When I left my dorm room the next morning—I promise you—I was a different person with a new goal.

Deciding to Change

In general, the experience made me a more motivated person. In the next few years after that day, I would graduate, climb the ranks at my work, get a promotion, and finish an MBA program. The kind of motivation and determination that came over me that night was like nothing else I've experienced, before or after.

The moment I got back to my dorm room, I knew I wasn't the same anymore. That moment spun me around, and I found myself in a full sprint heading in the other direction. It's crazy because it wasn't anything very dramatic: It was a completely normal day. I didn't have a crisis; it wasn't like I tripped and suddenly realized, "Oh wait, I shouldn't be fat." It was the same day I'd had a hundred times before, this time with a completely new perspective on life. I had stayed stagnant in my habits and confidence for nineteen years, and suddenly I was seeing myself in a new light. I thought, "My life could be completely different than it is now." It was the exact opposite of déjà vu: Instead of doing something new and feeling I had done it before, I followed my daily routine and felt it was unfamiliar to me. Something about it wasn't right. I wanted something better for myself, and I started to believe that I could achieve it.

Maybe it's the inner fat kid in me, but I liked to compare my new perspective on life to what people experience with food. You grow up eating your family's cooking—your mom, dad, or grandma's food—and you love it. Maybe your parents are great cooks, or maybe they're not; you don't know the difference because it's all you know. Whatever you eat feels normal to you; then as an adult, you order a Mac and Cheese from a new restaurant, and it's as if it's for the first time. You had no idea mac and cheese could be this good because you've been eating the same recipe your entire life! You didn't know this was an option—a better option—and now you want that new kind of mac and cheese all the time! You were totally content before with the old stuff; but now you know what's out there, and you can't go back.

I truly believe I will never get to that level of motivation again. It was a significant emotional event for me, and it carried me through the most difficult parts of this long process. All I could think about was losing weight and dedicating myself to my goals. I had no idea what to do, but I was going to do it, no matter what.

I'm very thankful to the girl at the grill. That moment changed my life for the better.

When people ask about the success of my weight loss, I resort to a cliché. I tell them, "It was just a lifestyle change." That's not entirely true. You don't just make a lifestyle change on a whim. That moment fueled my lifestyle change certainly—it was the internal shift that made the change successful. It wasn't so much the girl herself, but more so it was my realization about what I was missing. I couldn't do without it anymore. Something had to click for me, and something will click for you, too. You have to decide to pick yourself up and be a grown-up who gets shit done. You have to be the one who takes responsibility and hold yourself accountable. You have to want it.

I don't know how many people have tried to help you lose weight. If it's anything like mine, my guess is that the number is high. If they haven't gone through the process themselves, though, they might not stress this point enough: You have to have a reason you want to lose weight.

This goes back to what I've said about your "reason why." I really want you to understand this point. A reason is different than just hype and willpower. Motivation alone will not get you where you want to be. That kind of endless motivation does not exist. That's why not many people can accomplish this. Weight loss programs and personal trainers may say they can give you everything you need, but they're wrong. If everything is external, you're going to lose steam when it really starts to matter.

You have to decide your reasons for pursuing a healthy life. It could be positive: something you are pursuing or working towards, negative: something you want to avoid at all costs, or even that you want to become healthy for your current spouse. Maybe you think of your children: You want to stay alive and active for your kids and your grandkids. Perhaps you want to become more attractive to get the chance to reject the people who shunned you before. Your reason doesn't matter to me, as long as it matters to you.

Your "reason why" will make all the difference for you. A switch flips in your mind and, with that, failure is no longer an option. This mindset applies to any difficult goal you are trying to achieve. A change happens in your attitude, and you know you're going to get to the finish

A switch flips in your mind and, with that, failure is no longer an option

line—whether it's getting through high school, graduating from college, starting a business, getting married, or getting a promotion. You see this kind of determination in the music industry. Some of the most famous people in the industry came from straight up nothing. To their fans, it might seem like they became successful overnight, when they heard their song on the radio. If you hear an interview from one of them, you'll see that they had to hustle for years before anyone knew their names. Even with their talent, it was years before anyone paid attention to them. That didn't stop them; they kept at it and turned their careers into success stories. That doesn't happen from a whim of motivation. It starts with your drive until it's not just an option anymore—it's the only way you see yourself living.

Once you've found your reason, write it down, tape it up on your fridge. Write it on your mirror. Frame it, collage it, or make it a daily reminder on your phone. Do whatever you need to do to focus on it every day. You will hit a point where letting yourself slip just a little doesn't sound that bad. When binge eating and skipping the workout sounds like heaven. You'll have a shit day, and you'll want to reach for the candy. It's in those moments that you need to remind yourself why it's not worth it.

This time nothing was going to get in the way of my goal. Realistically, I'm sure that many factors in my life had prepared me for this change. If I hadn't found internal motivation, I don't think I would have been able to lose all that weight.

AARON KNIPP

The possibility of a relationship with that one particular girl was beside the point for me. It wasn't her, specifically, who motivated me to change: it was an idea. It was the idea that my size was preventing me from a potential future—a future I wanted and deserved! My weight was hindering me from having confidence to start a relationship and, by extension, keeping me from finding my future wife and having kids— something I'd always wanted for myself, a family of my own. My weight was keeping me from voicing my own opinions, wearing what I wanted to wear, and introducing myself to new people. My weight was pushing me down a spiral of insecurity. I was tired of the pain of people's rejection and disgust. I was tired of the judgment and insecurity. I was tired of not getting what I wanted or to where I wanted to go. I didn't want to feel tired anymore; I wanted to feel whole!

I focused on that idea every day, and that's what kept me going.

> I focused on that idea every day, and that's what kept me going

Unfortunately, while internal motivation is essential, it's not the only thing you'll need. All the motivation in the world cannot make up for the right tools. For me, researching about weight loss became a compulsion. After staying up that one night on my laptop, I spent hours each day learning more. My journey was not a perfect one, but in the end I achieved what I needed. To finally get to a good place in my health, it took me years. I'd do well for a couple of months, fall off my routine for a week, I'd get on track again, and then I'd mess up some more. As

34

the months went on, I gained knowledge and became even more efficient at losing weight, and falling out of my routine became less common.

Next, I'm going to lay out the plan that helped me lose the weight: what I ate, my exercises, and how I spent my day. I'll tell you what worked and what didn't work. I'll save you the months of wasted time by warning you about what I wish someone had told me. I've said it already that I *always* try to find the easiest way to do things. This is it. So let's get you started!

CHAPTER FOUR

Calories in, Calories Out

'm going to start with what worked for me: the plan that really effected change. Even today, I follow this plan. I'll move to exercise and how burning calories works in this system soon after. Once we have an understanding of how it works, I'll detail my daily and weekly routines before sharing tips on how to succeed and what to avoid. In all of this, my hope is that you will find a sustainable and effective rhythm for your life. I want you to save time and get the body you want a little faster. It all starts with understanding the basics.

Basal Metabolic Rate

Calories are energy for the body. They are what allows you to walk around, exercise, and do everyday tasks. Even without running around, your body requires a certain number of calories each day to have enough energy to keep everything running smoothly.

The number of calories required to maintain your particular body is called a 'Basal Metabolic Rate' or BMR

Your car needs gas, your smartphone needs a battery, and the human body needs calories. These basic functions are not optional: breathing, pumping blood through your body, fighting disease, producing waste, etc. The number of calories required to maintain your particular body is called a "Basal Metabolic Rate" or BMR. Everyone has a different BMR, depending on size.

Very simply, when you eat more calories than your BMR allows, then you gain weight, because your body stores the extra calories it doesn't use. Likewise, if you eat fewer calories than your BMR number, you lose weight. Your body finds the calories it needs in your stored fat.

There are 3,500 calories in a pound. This means that in order to gain one pound, you need to incorporate an extra 3,500 calories into your diet. This could be over a month, a week, or even a day—depending on how much you are over-eating. In order to lose one pound, 3,500 calories will need to be deducted from your BMR number. Say you eat 500 calories less than your BMR: 500 less per day over the course of a week translates to one pound lost. Over the course of a month, you will lose four pounds. If you consume 1000 calories less per day than your BMR, then you are looking at a weight loss of two pounds per week and eight pounds per month.

Let's say your BMR is 2,000. For you to maintain your current weight, you can eat 2,000 calories each day. Hypothetically, if you eat 2,500 calories a day (and don't exercise), you are over your allowance by 500 calories each day, which is 3,500 calories in a week. At this rate, you are gaining one pound each week (3,500 calories per seven days). However, if you eat 1,500 calories a day (still without exercise), you are under your BMR by 500 calories a day, which totals to 3,500 calories lost in a week. You will lose one pound a week (3,500 calories).

I spent months researching my weight loss and healthy living questions. I also reached out to friends who were in shape: my roommate at the time, who was studying nutrition, and another buddy pursuing bodybuilding. I'd steal my roommate's nutrition study book off his desk and look up information. I'd ask others for their gym tips. Honestly, I asked everyone around me questions—as many questions as I could think of. I also went to professionals: I paid for personal training, and I enrolled in a nutrition class too.

I did all this research on my own: I do not have any official certifications. At the end of the day, though, my greatest learning came from my own experience of trying and failing. I'm just a former fat kid who figured it out.

First, calculate your own BMR, Basal Metabolic Rate. Now pay attention, this is the most important number in this whole deal. I've listed the calculation below, but you can also look it up online. So let's stop and take a moment away from reading this book to go calculate your BMR. It will take you only a few seconds to look it up online.

So let's stop and take a moment away from reading this book to go calculate your BMR

BMR (Basal Metabolic Rate) Equation:

Women: BMR = 655 + (4.35 x weight in pounds) + (4.7 x height in inches) - (4.7 x age in years)

Men: BMR = 66 + (6.23 x weight in pounds) + (12.7 x height in inches) - (6.8 x age in years)

Okay, now you know how many calories it takes for you to stay exactly where you are. This information—this number lodged in your head—is so valuable. Even if you hate me and don't finish this book, or even if you just don't want to start your weight loss right now, at least you know your BMR. You know the number of calories it takes to keep you at the same weight and honestly, even if you aren't trying, I bet subconsciously you'll be more aware of the calories you consume. You may even unknowingly cut back a little now that you have this information. Knowledge is the tool, execution is power, and you cannot make informed decisions about your eating patterns unless you know your BMR.

Your next step is to pick a time-specific weight loss goal. You might want to lose ten pounds in two months. Maybe you want to lose twenty-five pounds in three months. Calculate the calories and divide by your time frame. I suggest using small time frames: one week or one month. Say you want to lose ten pounds in one month. Multiply ten by 3,500 to calculate total calories, then divide it by thirty to know how many calories you need to lose each day.

(10 pounds x 3,500 calories) / 30 = 1,167 calories each day.

Say your BMR is 2,700. Then subtract 1,167 from 2,700 to know how many calories you need each day: 1,533.

I like to think of this number as my daily calorie allowance.

Equation for Daily Calorie Allowance:

BMR - [(Weight to lose in pounds x 3,500 calories) / Days of time frame goal] = **Daily Calorie Allowance**

It really is this easy. All these commercial diets and all the websites will have you believe that they have the secret to weight loss. They don't, but now you do. This is what it takes, and I wish I would've known this from the beginning. If you want to lose one pound in a week, then your calorie allowance is 500 under your BMR. If you want to lose three pounds a week, your calorie allowance is 1,500 under your BMR. Your calorie allowance is the other important number to lock in your mind during your weight loss journey. Your BMR tells you what you need to **stay** where you are. Your calorie allowance gives what you need to **aim** for to lose weight. I call the number of calories you lose your deficit. If your calorie allowance is 1,500 and your BMR is 2,000, then your deficit for the day (if you stick to eating 1,500 calories) is 500.

To implement this system, you'll need to look up the caloric value of your food. There are so many different apps and websites that will do this for you. With modern technology, you can simply Google how many calories an avocado has. You have the information at your fingertips: *Use it*! Sure, it may be annoying to look up everything you're eating all the time, but it soon becomes second nature. I've been doing this for so long that I have many meals memorized, or, if I do not have the specific item memorized, I can provide myself a pretty accurate guess. Off the top of my head, I can tell you how many calories are in a chicken sandwich and how many calories in a slice of pepperoni pizza. At first, it's a chore to constantly look up everything you eat. After a few months of making it a habit, you'll start to have an idea of what something is before you even pick up your phone. I'll go more in depth about this in my chapter on routines, but I can tell you right now that you will probably find your favorite low-calorie meals and stick to those foods. (Turn

NEVER go below 1200 calories a day

to the back of the book for examples of some of my favorite foods.)

Seeing how many calories you'll intake in a day is a big shock. Before I started losing weight, I was consuming about 5,500 calories a day, easily. My BMR at that time was about 2,860, so I was eating 2,640 over my allowance and gaining over five pounds in a week. I was not doing myself any favors. This was not a good path to health.

The implementation piece takes a trial period. How big you are and what kind of diet you want to maintain influences how ambitious or moderate your weight loss goals can be. Pick

42

a goal, then stick to it for one to two weeks before adjusting. Everyone's pace and goals will be different. We all start from a different place. Everyone has a unique body and lifestyle and healthy looks different on everyone. I'm not here to tell you what your goal needs to be: I'm here to empower you to plan your own way to a healthier life.

Using BMR to build a weight loss plan relies on the science of losing weight by calorie regulation. However, there are a few important facts to remember as you sketch out your goals and begin implementing them:

1. Not all weight loss is fat loss. For the first few weeks of your plan, you might see extra weight fall off due to water weight and non-essential "gunk" that is just sitting in your body. When you start managing your diet, your body will recognize that you are trying to make a healthy change and will start to flush out all of the extras. Obesity makes you carry all kinds of nonsense in your body. Time to be rid of it.

   Pick a goal, then stick to it for one to two weeks before adjusting

2. After a significant amount of weight is lost, you might experience a plateau. It's important to remember this does not last forever. It's just a speed bump. All this means is that your body fell into the routine of losing weight and is now somewhat immune to your weight loss strategy. This is your chance to take it to the next level, adapt. Add something else in: up your walk from

thirty to forty-five minutes or lower your calorie intake. You're ready for another challenge.

3. Your BMR is based on your weight and whether you are male or female. This means, as you lose large quantities of weight, your BMR will change. As you lose five or ten pounds, recalculate your calorie allowance, look to new target goals, and proceed.

Essentially, the more you exercise, the more you can eat!

4. Some people go to extremes to lose weight and might fall into starvation mode. Starvation mode is when you eat too few calories throughout the day and your body cannot run its everyday activities. Side effects include hair loss, fatigue, and muscle loss. I cannot stress this enough: **NEVER** go below 1200 calories a day. Even though your body pulls from fat to get calories, it cannot strictly pull from fat without sending your body emergency signals. You need a constant flow of calories. You need to eat every day. Do not send your body into emergency mode.

5. So far, I have only addressed weight loss given a sedentary lifestyle. Your BMR meets you at your very laziest: the amount of calories you need to lie in bed all day. Many people—especially those who are overweight— do not incorporate exercise into their lives. That is fine—you do not have to. As I explained, as long as you

keep track of your caloric intake and keep to your plan, you will lose weight. However, the amount of exercise you get greatly influences how many daily calories you can have. This final point leads me to the last step in my basic weight loss plan. You factor in exercise.

How Exercise Saved My Ass

Now that you have your BMR, we are ready to get going! Just to recap, if you eat more calories than your daily allowance, then you gain weight. If you eat fewer calories than your BMR, you create a deficit, and you lose weight. In the allowance system, you use your BMR to calculate your daily calorie allowance, based on how many pounds you want to lose in a set period of time.

I want to stress: I know this is a lot of information thrown to you at one time—but I promise you, you've got this! You have your BMR, your calorie allowance, and you might have even started looking up a couple of food items to check out their caloric value. If so, I know what you're thinking: "Seriously . . . my caloric allowance is SO LOW." And you're totally right. It is low. And once you start comparing calorie allowance to actual calories in foods which you love to eat, you'll see that you don't have much room to work with. That allowance gets used up fast! Say your daily allowance is 1,500 calories. If you eat a bagel sandwich for breakfast and have fast food for lunch, you're already out of calories for the day.

But there is hope. So far, I have been strictly speaking

for a person who does not exercise. Many of us live sedentary lifestyles. If we are students or have a desk job, the only walking in our lives may be from our houses to our cars. When you are obese, the temptation to sit and rest becomes even more compelling. As I described before, even walking across the street strains your body, making you sweat. Your BMR number is the number of calories you need to stay at the same weight, without doing any exercise—just living your life as average—and, as we've covered, your calorie allowance is based off of this number, and your deficit is the difference between the two.

Exercise allows you to increase your calorie allowance or increase your deficit. Essentially, the more you exercise, the more you can eat! If you want to eat more than your calorie allowance, you can always hit the gym or go on a walk. If you exceed your allowance faster than anticipated, you can go on a run to gain it back. If you are doing well and want to get ahead of your own schedule, losing weight even faster, you can go to a gym class. There are so many modern tools you can use to track your exercise: Online calculators or fitness monitors will tell you how many calories you are burning. Remember, whatever you burn you get back for the day!

Personally, there have been so many times where exercise has saved my ass. I have been in each of these scenarios below, and, each time, exercise has been my lifeline. You'll face these situations too! Let me describe them for you.

Scenario One

Let's say that a man—we'll call him Terry—is using my allowance system to lose weight. He has a BMR of 2,000 calories. In order to lose one pound a week, his daily allowance is 1,500 calories (deficit of 500 calories each day). Terry is doing really well so far. He's kicking ass, eating exactly what he's supposed to, and he's been on track all week. But when he wakes up Sunday morning, he wakes up with a huge craving for pancakes.

So Terry decided to go to brunch with a few friends. After a few hours, what could have been a light brunch turns into bottomless mimosas with French toast and bacon. In just one meal, Terry has consumed 1600 calories! Well, this isn't good news for Terry because not only did he go over his daily calorie allowance, but it's only 1:30 in the afternoon! He's looking at an entire afternoon and evening without eating anything else! He's run out of calories for the day—from 1:30 to midnight, he can't have food. He knows he's screwed. Even though he's been doing so well this week, he thinks of giving up. He's blown it at brunch.

This is where exercise can be a game changer. Instead of giving up on life and gaining back the weight, Terry can exercise. He can hit the gym for an hour to burn a few hundred calories. He can go on a walk, he can take a hike, or he can even just take laps around the mall! Terry has options. As long as he

exercise can be a game changer

47

tracks what he burns, he gains flexibility on his calorie allowance for the day.

He decides to go on an hour walk, and he burns 400 calories. Now, instead of being at 1600 for the day, he gets to subtract 400. Now he is only at 1200! Because he is under his allowance for the day, he has 300 calories available for a light dinner later when he gets hungry. If Terry doesn't want a light meal and, instead, wants a 600-calorie bowl of cereal for dinner, he can have that! He can go on another forty-five-minute walk, burn about 300 more calories, and he's golden! Terry is right on track. No need to throw it all away because he wanted to enjoy himself. It's all about finding a balance that works for you.

Scenario Two

Alternatively, exercise can also help you lose more pounds in a week. Let's take Terry as an example again. He has a BMR of 2,000, and he's still going for an allowance of 1,500 calories a day. He's on track to lose one pound a week, and he's been keeping to it. He listened to Aaron and stopped eating everything in sight because he didn't need to. He's looking up the caloric value of his food, and he's been so consistent in keeping to his allowance that he's now within eight pounds of where he wants to be.

But Terry has a new problem on his hands. He just agreed to a vacation with his family. This vacation is in one month, and this timing is screwing up Terry's plan. One pound each week only affords him four pounds. That rate just isn't going to cut it because his family is going on a cruise, and he wants to look really good. Instead of losing only four pounds in the next month, he'd like to double that number and lose the entire eight.

Hypothetically, what he wants to do is lower his calorie allowance and increase his deficit Based on his BMR of 2,000, his current allowance is at 1,500, with a 500 deficit. Doubling his deficit takes him from an allowance of 1,500 to an allowance of 1,000!

This simply isn't going to be enough food for Terry. Eating only 1000 calories a day puts a person in starvation mode, and starvation mode damages the body. Terry would start to lose hair and find himself to be irritable and uncontrollably hungry. What Terry can do is keep his daily allowance at 1,500 calories and incorporate an extra 500 calories of exercise into his daily routine. With that fix, he'll be able to lose two full pounds each week and look really good for his cruise.

Scenario Three

Unlike the binge eating in scenario one or the accelerated, vacation-oriented goal of scenario two, scenario three is about everyday modifications. Again, imagine that Terry would like to eat 1,500 calories a day. His BMR is 2,000. However, each day he finds himself slipping from his goal: not in big ways, but just by a little bit. He finds himself hungry throughout the day and craving snacks. He picks healthy snacks—fruit and power bars—but they still add too much to his overall calories for the day. He keeps tallying up at about 1,700 calories a day.

This frustrates Terry. He feels that he's doing everything he can to be conscious of his food intake, and he doesn't want to give up snacks or lunch. While he's still losing weight (he's under his BMR), he's not sticking to his goals. He can't seem to shave off that last 200 calories from his diet: he gets too hungry, and the food he wants to eat simply has too many calories to fit into his plan.

This is when incorporating small, daily workouts can be so helpful to this process. If Terry decides to walk every day or literally to get on the stationary bike for thirty minutes and stream Netflix, he can keep on track. This is not about a crazy weekend binge and then hitting the gym hardcore to make up for it. This is measured, small doses of burning calories. If Terry can't fit in a workout every day, he could, instead, schedule more sustained workouts three or four times a week.

For most people, what works best is a combination of both exercise and food monitoring. If you know you can maintain a 1,700-calorie lifestyle but your calorie allowance is 1,400, then use exercise to make up the difference. It's all about developing a healthy rhythm. Especially if your BMR is near the 1,200-calorie starvation-mode mark, then exercise can help you get the food your body needs for the day as well as continue to lose some of the excess weight.

With that being said, it will take a few weeks for you to get in a routine. You'll probably try something out each week and you'll tweak it just a little until you are completely comfortable with the amount you eat, exercise, and lose. What's important is that you find something sustainable. Anyone is capable of sticking to a diet program for a couple of days, but if you are going to make a big change in your size, then you need to be able to commit for months. You can't kill yourself by over-exercising or starving yourself living on baby carrots. If you absolutely need a hamburger, plan that into your point system. If you just have to binge one weekend, then plan to make up the difference. The key is consistency.

I will not lie to you. Consistency is difficult. It took me two years to lose 140 pounds, but I could have done that in less time had I committed to a plan. Even though I'm healthy now, and I don't need to lose significant weight, I still use the point system. I still measure what I need to eat and what I need to lose to stay on track. I still adjust for vacations and splurges. I have made a habit of going to the gym and incorporating exercise into my daily routine. What's amazing is that, now, I actually look forward to working out. The best part of my day is going to lift weights. I promise—I never thought that I could feel that way. Working out was not my thing, but it became part of my day. It wasn't easy, but I found a sustainable rhythm that works for me, one in which I keep track of what I eat and exercise. Better yet, it gave me the ability to eat the food I actually want to eat and still lose and maintain the weight!

The key is consistency.

Next, I'll share the rhythms that worked for me—the easiest possible way I've found.

CHAPTER FIVE

Wake Up, Show Up, Repeat

The absolute hardest thing in the world is just to keep it up. The easiest way I know to keep it up is to commit to a routine. Think of your day-to-day now. You do the same things typically, right? So why not commit yourself to a new routine that benefits you. Once you show up, all you have to do is go through the motions. Once you make new habits, you're set.

Old Rhythms

I used to be full for months. When you eat a complete meal (with dessert) every three or four hours, you never feel hunger.

With a daily caloric intake of 5,000- 6,000 calories, I was taking on weight at an aggressive pace: five pounds a week

When I was in college, I had access to an unlimited amount of food. Here is what a typical day would look like:

At about 10:30 a.m., I'd wake up and head over to the student union. I'd start with a bowl of cereal (300 calories). I loved drinking vitamin water—which has lots of sugar—with three to four refills. Three drinking cups of that would give me another 300 calories. Since it was close to noon, I'd treat this first meal like a brunch rather than breakfast. I'd get a cheeseburger and fries (300 for the fries, 270 for the bun, and 200 calories for two pieces of cheese, and then 300 for the meat).

Later in the day, I'd go for an 800-calorie burrito and, again, three refills of whatever I was drinking—Gatorade this time (150). For dinner, I'd often get an off-brand Panda Express meal, since that was available to me on campus. That's another 1,700-calorie meal right there. Then, as I described before, I'd go with my friends for a fourth meal. We'd head over to Taco Bell at about 10:00 p.m., and we'd down another 1,500 calories in burritos. If we didn't decide to go to Taco Bell, we'd at least get Frozen Yogurt at the student union, which is another 1,000 calories. If we were feeling up to it, we'd do both.

At 320 pounds, my BMR was 2,858. With a daily caloric intake of 5,000–6,000 calories, I was taking on weight at an aggressive pace: five pounds a week. Because this was my routine, it's what I did without thinking. It was my go-to.

Trying to lose weight required a huge shift in these patterns. When I wanted to go for another refill or a fourth meal, I had to tell myself no. When I didn't know what food to eat, it was very tempting to fall back into my previous habits.

What I needed was a new set of habits and new routines. I needed a new autopilot. When I didn't have a set plan, when I shifted to a new plan, or when I tried something different, these were the times I was likely to mess up. Sometimes, I'd crave my old habits and slip up. Other times, I was just bored of eating the same few foods, and I'd change up my schedule for no reason at all. Either way, I found myself getting off-course from my goals.

Sticking to a routine is invaluable for your weight loss journey. It is so important. It will take you a few weeks for you to get down the foods you like, the exercise you can tolerate, what times you eat, how many times you eat—all that good stuff. You'll see the difference between a bowl of chips and a bowl of spaghetti. You'll be surprised by the healthy snacks, which actually have more calories than unhealthy ones. This education is the difficult part, so give yourself grace for finding those meals that satisfy you and work for your plan. Like many people, I now have about seven favorite meals that I routinely eat. But don't let yourself off the hook: there's a difference between figuring out what works for you and simply changing a plan because you are bored. When you finally find something that works for you, try to stick with it.

The process of changing your lifestyle is hard, and this autopilot thing is going to be a lifesaver for you! Something that helped me a lot, especially in the beginning, was downloading an app to track my calories. That way, I had a resource with me at all times. It was super convenient and kept me on track. There are going to be so many times when you are out and about and you might not know the

Sticking to a routine is invaluable for your weight loss journey

calories in a certain food, or you guess on how many calories you burned during a specific exercise. An app makes it so easy to look up calorie information and keep a record of what you eat. I cannot recommend it enough.

Let's be real with each other: I can't think of a single person who doesn't have habits—with their meals or activities—that shape their everyday life. Without a routine that works for you, you'll struggle. Please don't make this more difficult than it needs to be. Pick your foods, pick your exercises, and just continue to kick ass in the most mundane way every single day!

A Week in My Weight Loss Life

When I was just starting out on my weight loss journey, I read different strategies and testimonies about how to lose weight. The people and programs always provided a plan of what to eat for the day. None of these meal plans were realistic for me. They all took a similar pattern. Something like this:

- Breakfast: two egg whites and some oatmeal
- Snack: protein drink
- Lunch: grilled chicken and rice
- Dinner: something gross that I never actually wanted to eat

My immediate reaction was, "What the hell is this?" Whoever thought that I, Aaron, could stick to that plan for the rest of my life was full of it. Had the creators of these diets tried their own plans? They believed lettuce, egg whites, and a "fun" three-mile walk would magically make losing weight a blast. They were "super excited" for this fat guy to get on their plan. Technically, their plan would make me lose weight—but, damn, it would suck eating like that every day, forever. Honestly, it's naive to imagine that someone as large as I was could buy into that kind of eating and stick to it.

> They believed lettuce, egg whites, and a "fun" three-mile walk would magically make losing weight a blast

What I want to do is walk you through an actual week of mine. I want to emphasize this was a legitimate week for me. I'm not going to exaggerate or substitute information to make it look better. I'm going to use specific food places and specific meals. I cannot say that this food is healthy or that the portions are perfect. I only mean to provide real examples of what I ate when I was losing weight. I'm doing this not only to give you a good idea of how realistic this weight loss plan is, but also so you can see I'm a real person who eats crap sometimes—but who was still able to lose weight.

Example Week:

Monday:
- Breakfast: Greek yogurt - 80 calories
- Lunch: Chipotle burrito - roughly 1,100 calories (half-serving white rice, half-serving black beans, double chicken, cheese, sour cream, pico sauce, lettuce)

- Dinner: Greek yogurt - 80 calories
- Late night snack: muscle milk, light - 110 calories
- Exercise: one-hour weight lifting - 500 calories burned

Calories consumed: 1,370

Calories burned: 500

Calorie total for the day: 870

Tuesday:
- Breakfast: protein shake - 150 calories
- Lunch: In-N-Out Double-Double cheeseburger with fries - roughly 1,200 calories
- Dinner: Peanut butter and jelly sandwich - 450 calories
- Exercise: one-hour weight lifting - 500 calories burned

Calories consumed: 1,800

Calories burned: 500

Calorie total for the day: 1,300

Wednesday:
- Breakfast: skip
- Lunch: Chick-fil-A nuggets, 12 count - 400 calories
- Dinner: Cane's six-strip combo with sauce, fries, and an Arnold Palmer - roughly 1,800 calories
- Exercise: one-hour weight lifting - 500 calories burned

Calories consumed: 2,200

Calories burned: 500

Calorie total for the day: 1,700

Thursday:
- Breakfast: breakfast burrito of three eggs, cheese, and hash browns - 850 calories
- Lunch: protein bar - 200 calories

- Dinner: Chick-fil-A, nuggets, 12 count - 400 calories
- Exercise: none

Calories consumed: 1,450

Calories burned: 0

Calorie total for the day: 1,450

Friday:

- Breakfast: Greek yogurt - 80 calories
- Lunch: Peanut butter and jelly sandwich - 450 calories
- Dinner: Cane's six-strip combo with sauce, fries, and an Arnold Palmer - roughly 1,800 calories
- Exercise: one-hour weight lifting 500 calories burned

Calories consumed: 2,330

Calories burned: 500

Calorie total for the day: 1,830

Saturday:

- Breakfast: Greek yogurt - 80 calories
- Lunch: homemade burrito (chicken, rice, black beans, cheese) - roughly 800 calories
- Dinner: chicken quesadilla - 700 calories
- Late night snack: Greek yogurt - 80 calories
- Exercise: one-and a half-hour of weight lifting - 750 calories burned

Calories consumed: 1,660

Calories burned: 750

Calorie total for the day: 910

Sunday:

- Breakfast: breakfast burrito of three eggs, cheese, hash browns - 850 calories

- Lunch: chicken quesadilla - 700 calories
- Dinner: four eggs and cheese - 400 calories
- Exercise: one-and-a-half-hour of weight lifting - 750 calories burned

Calories consumed: 1,950

Calories burned: 750

Calorie total for the day: 1,200

That's an example of a week for me. Some weeks, I'll go on a weird streak of eating Chipotle five times in a row, and other times I'll have nothing but quesadillas and breakfast burritos all week. You can clearly see that I didn't eat a single damn salad. Not only did I avoid tasteless salads, I ate all the same food that I was eating when I was severely overweight.

I didn't eat a single damn salad

Let's pause for a second. I really want you to see the difference in what I'm suggesting compared to what the weight loss programs say. I've seen so many infomercials which advertise weight loss pills/food plans where they say they are giving you "all of your favorite foods" and still lose weight. A thin person in activewear will face the camera and say, "I lost eighty pounds while eating food I love!" The camera pans to a shitty-looking "healthy" pizza that you know tastes like cardboard. Hell no. I seriously ate like a fifteen-year-old, and, as long as I kept under the calories for the day, I lost weight.

Let's go through how this week of food affected my weight. In the recorded week, I totaled 12,760 calories. That averages out to about 1,822 calories a day. I burned a total of 3,500 calories through exercise which is an average of about 500 a day. If my BMR was 2,000, then my calorie total would make a deficit of 678 for the day, and 4,740 for the week! That's 2,000 minus my calorie intake plus the calories I burned. This is how much I'm taking off each day, which totals to be 4,746 a week! That 4,746 translates into 1.35 pounds. I lost 1.35 pounds while eating fried chicken and breakfast burritos.

I want to make this crystal clear to you because it's really important that you see how feasible this plan is. This week, I ate fast food—a lot of it every day this week—and I still lost almost a pound and a half. I did go to the gym, but I only gave an average effort and didn't stay for more than an hour and a half. I still lost about a pound and a half. This is without trying very hard.

> I lost 1.35 pounds while eating fried chicken and breakfast burritos

I've told you that I like finding the easiest way to do things. That was how I went about school, how I got through my nine-to-five job, and how I lost 140 pounds. Losing weight is hard enough without any extra complications! I don't want to ever have to give up the foods I like. I definitely don't want any of the bullshit where I have to wait two weeks to eat half of a chicken strip. Seriously, it really doesn't get any easier than this! I ate "unhealthy" every day and still lost weight. Why? Because I've found balance in eating what I love and still being healthy Trust me, if there was an easier way, I would have found it. This is it.

I can tell you how calories work, I can explain how exercise plays into losing weight, and even give you specific numbers on what I eat every day, but you're the one who has to start trying. Without your effort, these figures are just numbers on a page. Every new endeavor has a learning curve, and there will always be hiccups you cannot predict. When you start on your weight loss journey, it's just hard to anticipate what the day is going to throw at you. I can give you all the information you need, and you can be super pumped to get started, but you may still find that it takes time to get into a rhythm. The meal you prepared might not taste as great as you hoped, groceries might be more expensive than you anticipated, or maybe you counted on the gym being open until midnight and it closed at 9:30 p.m. in the evening. It could be anything. There are a million things that could go wrong in a day—especially when you are trying out new habits. My point is that it may take some time to get used to your new schedule. Give yourself grace and keep pushing! You are worth the challenge, and you are capable of making a commitment to yourself. You owe it to yourself to try!

A Day in My Weight Loss Life

The day-to-day looked really similar to the weekly routine. I really think that the trick to success is finding a routine you like and one to which you can commit. Some of this process just isn't going to be fun, so I encourage you to make it as painless for yourself as possible: find a routine.

Here is what my life looked like on an average weekday:

- **7:30–8:00 a.m.:** I woke up, made my bed, and prepared for the gym. Someone suggested once that I search why to make your bed in the morning. It sounded strange to me at the time, but I was eventually curious enough to check it out. And I was convinced—not only by what I found on the internet but also from my experience of trying it out. Making your bed in the morning does actually make a difference in your motivation for the day. When I made the effort to make my bed right away, I immediately took on a motivated mindset: I knew I wasn't getting back into bed. I was more motivated to get into my workout clothes, take my pre-workout, and go to the gym. Making my bed and taking the pre-workout before I walked out the door almost forced me not to walk my tired ass back right back into bed.

- **8:00–9:30 a.m.:** This was my gym time. I spent the first hour just lifting weights. Lifting weights is not everyone's favorite way to exercise. Personally, I like the way I feel when I lift and find it way better than jogging. After the first hour, if I felt like I needed to burn more calories, I jumped on the bike or the elliptical. Typically, I did not stay longer than twenty minutes more at the gym. I'd pull up a video to watch on my phone to help pass the time.

- **9:30–10:30 a.m.:** I went home, had a Greek yogurt, and relaxed for a bit. Everyone relaxes differently, but I relaxed by watching TV. I sat on my couch and watched more videos on YouTube for fifteen to twenty minutes. After that, it was time to get ready for the day, and I was out the door by 10:10 a.m. on my way to work.

- **Noon:** Midday meant snack time! It wasn't anything too big. I ate a protein bar, a shake—or maybe even a candy bar if it was offered to me. Whatever it was, I tried to keep my snacks under 300 calories.

- **3:00 p.m.:** Lunch time. For me, lunch is the biggest meal of the day. My snack got me through a couple hours of work, but I was hungry from my workout earlier in the day. Honestly, lunch was the only thing I usually thought about from the time I walked into work until three o'clock. Usually, it was a Chipotle or Chick-fil-A trip; the Chick-fil-A was within walking distance, so I'd strolled over there and used the extra calories burned for more chicken nuggets!

- **8:00 p.m.:** I'd be home from work at this time, and I might . . . MIGHT . . . if I had any calories left from my three o'clock meal, eat yogurt or something small. More than likely, the second I get home I changed into sweatpants and jumped in bed, so I could wind down for the day with my favorite Netflix shows.

- **11:00 p.m.:** If I hadn't already fallen asleep, I turned out the light.

That was it. I followed this routine every day during the week. It's what allowed me to keep my balance on those days I wasn't working. Describing what my average weekend looked like is a little more difficult. Sometimes I'd work out three times on a Saturday, and, in between workouts, I'd be super productive! I'd do laundry, eat healthy, and cross off all of my to-do items. Other times, I'd make ten bad decisions in a row. I was in my early twenties, so I still went out to eat, drink, and do things that weren't ideal for my health. I'd still put garbage in my body. So it depended on the weekend.

Weekends present lots of social opportunities, and social opportunities almost always involve food. I like to call these foods PWGs—potential weight gainers! A PWG is any food that is high in calories and unhealthy for you. Routine is so important during the week, so you can handle the PWGs when you choose to eat them. Splurging on the weekends (PWGs) is necessary—for a birthday or a special event—and sometimes you blink, and you just consumed 2,000 calories in a tequila and Mexican food. Other weekends will be opportunities to kick ass and lose even more weight than normal! Weekends can go either way. Track the PWGs. Always keep track of what you're eating, and stick to your routine as much as possible, but don't be afraid to have a little fun.

Keeping the Weight Off

For me, keeping off the weight is a continuation of the same habits I made when I was trying to lose weight. It's all about consistency, about getting to the gym, and making it happen. Even though my overall goals are different, I still need to track my calories, do the math, and measure what I'm gaining and losing.

The biggest difference now is that I've taken the time to know my body. I know what my average fluctuation is (weight-wise), what I can handle, and what puts me in the danger zone. I've looked up so many meals that I have a pretty good idea of how many calories each meal is. This is one of the many positives of losing weight! You get to know your own limits and your own potentials. Certainly, I do not have to be as strict as I used to be, but I will never go back to eating 5,000 calories in a day without working out.

The biggest difference now is that I've taken the time to know my body

This system has also allowed me to continuously expand to new goals: muscle gain, strength building, and flexibility. I lean on my routines: my morning workout, my meal monitoring, and my point calculations. It keeps me in check, so I don't have to worry about falling back into my old habits. I've learned to eat healthier over the years, but I also know that doesn't mean depriving myself of the things I love. I can have the foods I want and still keep on track. It all comes back to consistency and putting in the small effort for the long-term gains.

CHAPTER SIX

Pitfalls

I decided to lose weight in December of 2012. I was 320 pounds. By September of 2014, I was down to 180. What is not reflected in that timeline is how long it took me to learn how to lose weight. As I've said, I had no one to teach me, and I made a lot of mistakes. The first seventy pounds took me one-and-a-half years.

How long did the second seventy pounds take me? Four to six months. One and a half years compared to a few months is an incredible difference. Once I had found what worked, applying it was easy. I figured out my calorie system. I committed to a plan, and I gained traction. I found an efficient and effective way to lose weight.

Before I figured out my rhythm, I learned through trial and error. I accomplished a lot not only by working on myself for years but also by helping others along the way. I've seen others make some of my mistakes as well. I don't want you to have to stumble through this process like I did. I've already given you my point system, but I also want to lay out the issues that kept me working way harder and way longer than the effort and time my weight loss goals actually required.

This is what to avoid.

Powdered Meals and Supplements

Some of the biggest mistakes I made early on revolved around my diet.

For instance, I used to eat powdered meals. I signed up for a plan that sent me packages of what looked like protein powder. You added water, put them in the microwave, and they would turn into pancakes. They were absolutely disgusting and left me hungry. But they were only 130 calories a pancake, and I would eat them religiously. For a while, I had them every day, multiple times a day.

Meal replacement powders never leave you feeling good. You're replacing the natural nutrition you get from food with something that meets your calorie requirement. Think of drinking a vegetable supplement in the morning and then only eating protein bars for the rest of the day. It will leave you feeling empty because your body needs something more. But I was willing to do whatever it took to lose weight. I knew that losing over 100 pounds wouldn't be easy, so I assumed that this powdery pancake was part of that process. I was just doing what I thought I needed to do.

I know now that I didn't have to eat those meals. I could have eaten real food. You can eat food you like and still lose weight. In fact, like I've emphasized before, eating too few calories puts you in starvation mode and will not help you lose consistent weight. Monitoring your calories (calories in vs. calories out) is more important than keeping a strict diet of gross supplement powders. For example, today I've already eaten twice, and it's not even noon. I had an omelet and a dark chocolate bar. I had cheese and a freakin' chocolate bar. I could have been eating like that back then, too, instead of depriving myself with powdered nothing!

This powdered meal season of my life is an example of a horrible tactic I tried for months. It was unnecessary and made me miserable. The powdered meals I bought were more expensive than they needed to be. I would have them four or five times a day—on top of other meals. I was spending $20 plus on food I hated in hopes of losing weight—when I could have lost weight eating food I liked.

Buying vitamin supplements falls in a similar category as powdered meals. Buying supplements was something I did for a period of time, and it cost me lots of cash without giving me much in return. At 125 pounds lost, I tried supplements, and I got to the point of taking thirteen different pills every single day. I was taking a pre-workout, calcium pills, energy supplements, recovery supplements, vitamin C, and tons of other pills. Just like dieting, finding the supplements that work for you takes time and balance. I do take supplements now, but I take only a few . . . not thirteen. I was spending $550 a month on supplements instead of investing in real food. Supplements are not your easy ticket to losing weight faster. I'll save you the money right now by telling you that.

It's more important to focus on what you're eating (actual food) than to stress over (and spend money) on supplements. There's a big difference between relying on supplements for meals and actually just giving your diet an extra boost ("supplementing" your real meals). As much as possible, it's my advice to stick to real foods, and eat what you want!

Undereating, Binging, Substituting

Eating powdered meals and taking supplements were two ways that "following a food plan" became unhelpful for me. When I help people train, they are always tempted to deviate from the food plan. Even if they are super motivated, it is really easy for them to justify an extra snack or skip the food they don't want to eat. They'll think they know what's better for them, I know this because I was the same way.

I was training someone the other day who ditched his food plan in favor of protein bars. He was trying to eat less in order to lose more pounds, but he put his body in starvation mode. He didn't end up losing more than a pound that week, and he starved himself. He thought he was pushing himself harder by skipping out on food. It doesn't work that way. If you eat too much, you don't lose weight, and if you eat too little your body goes into shut down mode. Binging, of course, doesn't help you lose weight, but neither does starving yourself! Finding a balance (calories in, calories out) is what will help you get far. Losing weight can seem crazy difficult and confusing, but it doesn't have to be. I'm here to teach you what works, and if that still doesn't cut it, I'm here to help personally.

Unmanageable Goals

Another mistake I made was failing to break up my goals into smaller chunks. I looked at my goals in terms of big weight, and, of course, I was trying to lose a lot of pounds. I was 320 pounds, and I wanted to lose as much weight as quickly as possible. I was thinking in terms of fifty-pound increments, one or two extra pounds either way did not seem like a big deal to me. So when faced with an extra meal at Taco Bell on a Saturday night, I caved. I was trying to lose fifty pounds, so what did it matter if I binged this week? I'd start all over next week.

I was thinking in terms of fifty-pound increments, one or two extra pounds either way did not seem like a big deal to me

Facing unmanageable goals also meant I spent way too many hours trying to burn off calories when I overate. I spent all day exercising. If I could walk to my next location, I did. I was always trying to stay on the move. I was still in school and even skipped my classes to go to the gym. I would text my friends and ask them to take notes for me or describe our speech class assignment, and I would disappear for the entire day. I used the treadmill at the gym to walk, and I would set up for the day. I would put it at the highest incline to get as much out of it as possible. I sometimes switched it up and used the stationary bike. I was pushing myself harder than I needed to and with no results. Not only was my goal unmanageable, but I was interfering with my everyday routine and losing that balance.

On one particular day, I woke up and decided to research how many miles it would take to hike the Grand Canyon's most popular trail. I found the mileage, and then set out for the gym. Just like the other days, I set myself up on the treadmill. But, this time, I was dedicated to walking that Grand Canyon trail. It was one of the craziest things I've done in an attempt to lose weight faster. It was boring and excruciating, but I wanted so much to lose weight that I was willing to do anything—even something dramatic like pretending to hike the Grand Canyon.

I do not recommend this strategy to anyone. It was grueling. I was at the gym eight hours each day. It was a full-time job. If I hadn't been in school, I do not know how I would have done it. I don't think I could do it again today. But I was so motivated that I was willing to cancel all of my plans and ignore many of my responsibilities to burn as many calories as possible. What came after? I would crash: I would binge from the hunger and gain back four of the five pounds I had lost that week.

Both of these issues were a result of unmanageably large goals. Ironically, I used my big goals to justify both killing myself at the gym all day and also to eat 6,000 calories at night.

I had to learn to think small to achieve big results in the

long run. I started making my goal ten pounds—just ten pounds. One week can make a hell of a difference towards or against ten pounds. If I lost three pounds, I made significant progress toward my goal of ten. If I gained six pounds, it felt like a setback, but I knew I was still capable of reaching my ten-pound goal. Thinking in terms of the next ten pounds kept me motivated: I made it from 260 to 250, or 240 to 230. Ten pounds was achievable for me.

Even now, if I take a big picture approach, it is easy to give myself shortcuts. There are days I just don't want to do it. Monday night, at midnight, I came back from a trip to California, and I had gained a full ten pounds. This Friday, I go on another trip—and I'll probably gain some weight on that as well! While I'm at home, though, I'm back to my day-to-day grind: Tuesday through Thursday I plan to work out, eat right, and follow my routine. It would be so easy for me to justify being lazy all week—to say, "Well, if I know I'm going on vacation, I can start my routine when I get back." I've used that excuse before, and it ends up costing me a lot. I won't allow myself to have that mentality again. Just because I gained a few pounds doesn't mean I need to set myself back even farther. If I'm aiming to stay within a smaller range, then those three days can make all the difference. That way, when I am on a trip and I want to indulge, I know I can.

I had to learn to think small to achieve big results in the long run

Once I understood this concept, I focused on that smaller, achievable goal, telling myself each day, "Just ten more

75

pounds!" The extra effort of losing the little pounds and going for little goals was the difference between seventy pounds in a year and a half or seventy pounds in four months. To this day, these smaller goals are what keep me at the weight I want to be.

With food, manageable goals translate as a sustainable diet.

I've tried all the weight loss tricks in the book. I've been on every plan, and I've tried every diet. One by one, they always managed to fail at keeping the results. It's not that these programs don't do what they say they will do. They will make you lose weight. If you follow them to the letter, that number on the scale will go down. That's not their problem. The issue is that they are not sustainable. You cannot eat only vegetables for the rest of your life. They will try to make their meal options sound attractive: "You can eat all the vegetables you want!" Well, shit, for me, that includes zero vegetables. I do not want a single vegetable. I'm healthy, and even now I can't remember the last time I wanted a carrot. I do not want a meal of a thousand baby carrots. If given the choice, I'd choose two bites of a chicken sandwich over a room full of salad every time. This kind of dieting will help someone who only needs to lose ten to fifteen pounds, but it can't turn a ship around. If you have a lifestyle of overeating, then baby carrots are not going to cut it.

Your social life plays a factor in making these "prepackaged food plans" and "salad only solutions" unrealistic goals. Dinner with friends is no longer an option: too much temptation and no approved foods on your strict diet. Normal activities don't allow for you to bring your own Tupperware of food into establishments. That's why you need to be on top of creating the diet that works for you, so you can go out with friends without the guilt.

I tried to limit myself only to "healthy" food for a while, and I always ended up binging later. I needed more than salads and smoothies to make my diet work. What I learned is that I needed to focus more on portion control and create healthy alternatives to my usual orders. I found you can always find something that fits your particular tastes; you just have to be willing to try. As long as I was on top of making a diet that worked for me, I could no longer use the excuse of "not liking healthy foods" to keep me from losing weight.

If you have a lifestyle of overeating, then baby carrots are not going to cut it

These are all common pitfalls, ones I had to experience myself to find alternatives, so I wouldn't end up back at square one. I hope these serve as warnings, so you can avoid the defeat I felt when I encountered them. You will face your own struggles on your journey, ones that maybe I haven't. Life will throw all kinds of bullshit your way; you just need to keep your head up and your eyes on the end goal: the best version of you.

CHAPTER SEVEN

Bullshit

Losing significant amounts of weight is an intense and grueling process. You are working so hard to change your life and be healthy, to change your routines and give yourself a real chance. The emotional and physical trials of this process are challenges enough in themselves.

I hate to say it, but there are more obstacles coming your way. Distractions and excuses will come at you from all angles—and, if your journey is anything like mine, you'll sometimes give into the pressure. It's so easy to get sidetracked by people around you telling you to skip the gym, or to go out for that late-night snack. I wasted so much time during the first year and a half of trying to lose weight due to wanting to hang out with friends rather than work out. I allowed my own insecurities to get in my head and derail me. On those bad days, it was hard to remember my reason why. I wasted time, physical energy, and emotional energy. I let other people and myself distract from my routines and

I wasted time, physical energy, and emotional energy

79

goals. I wish I could tell you that I kept on track—that I was able to shrug off what the world threw at me. But that's not the truth. It wasn't until the last part of my journey that I was able to breathe and block all of those other voices out. Before then, I was caught in the bullshit.

I am convinced that you will experience similar challenges, but I don't want you to have the same kind of setbacks I faced. With awareness, you can avoid this from the start.

Opinions

Honestly, I hate that I even have to address the issue of other people's opinions. It pains me to remember how much grief I let other people cause me during my weight loss process. Hands down, this was the number one struggle for me. I allowed my fear of what other people thought keep me down. I gave it the energy to fuel any lingering doubts I had.

Even though my friend knows a lot about fitness, his advice only distracted me from my goals

Some of the closest people to you don't realize that they are doing more harm than good. Some may think you're going to drop the lifestyle the same way you had any fad diet from before. They try to tell you what they think you should do or try to deter you from your path onto another because it will get you there faster. You are creating the pace for YOUR journey, not theirs, so remember to listen but also take it with a grain of salt. They are not in your shoes, they don't know what you want more than you. You are the only one with the power to change your mindset and lifestyle, so it goes without saying that you are the only one who can allow someone else's opinions to affect you. I say this because during the majority of my journey, I was weighed down by the opinions of others. I want better for you because it will help keep you focused on what matters.

Each person has a unique perspective, and each person believes their take is the best. People's opinions often contradict each other. You can't follow everyone's advice, even if you wanted to. You can't follow your friend Melissa's advice to eat a big breakfast and then nothing in the evening and simultaneously follow her boyfriend Mark's plan of a light breakfast and post-workout recovery meals. You can't live as a vegetarian at the same time as taking on a high-protein meat diet. You cannot stick to your own plan and follow every idea that Aunt Karen suggests for you at family gatherings.

To be fair, I believe that most people have good intentions. Chances are, the people who give you advice are your family and friends. They mean well, and they want to see you happy. With that in mind, I want you to be clear: the only one who knows what routine is best for you is yourself. I love my friends and family, and I've received lots of advice on my health over the years, but it was very overwhelming. I know they wanted the best for me, as your friends and family want the best for you. Just because they know you well doesn't mean they can grasp what your journey is going to be or what you're experiencing.

It's not their fault that they are unaware of your experience. How could they possibly know? The experience of being overweight—what you and I have to deal with on a daily basis—is unlike anything they have ever faced. They don't know what it's like to have strangers stare directly at you as you walk down the grocery aisle. They don't know what it's like to feel trapped in an endless cycle of eating poorly, feeling ashamed of yourself, and then eating poorly again in an effort to comfort yourself. For many of us, food is both the problem and what we use to try to fix the problem. I know what it feels like to have the only piece of control in your life be what is put in your body. If whoever throws advice at you has not been as big as you, then they simply cannot understand your life.

This journey is your own. Focus on that fact

This journey is your own. Focus on that fact. When you start your journey, when you commit to a rhythm of healthy decisions, when you start dropping weight every week like a badass—right then, right in the middle of your kickass rhythm, someone who loves you and means well will march right in and tell you what you're doing wrong.

Over the years, people have given me all kinds of ridiculous advice. When I was just starting out and getting into the groove of weight loss, I was working out every day. I wasn't used to restricting my eating, so I was working out to allow myself the food I wanted. One day, while shooting hoops at the gym for a few hours, my friend came up to me to tell me to stop. He said, "Man, I feel like all you do is focus on this weight loss stuff. You are doing too much, and it's probably unhealthy." Honestly, it was so discouraging to hear that. It made me feel like I wasn't allowed to try to be healthy. I was trying to figure out my routine, and this made me feel like I was doing it all wrong. Isn't that the point? I'm trying to find out what works for me, it doesn't happen overnight. I was finally getting some traction! I was finally dropping pounds! I was feeling better than I ever had in my life—and, yet, here he was, telling me I was unhealthy. It stopped me in my tracks.

Even now, even though I've reached a good point in my health, people tell me what to do. People love telling you how they would do your life. For example, my time at the gym has become my version of self-care. It's what makes me feel like I've accomplished something in my day. It is a part of my daily routine, and I look forward to my time there. Recently, while out with my parents for lunch, I mentioned heading to the gym. My mother, whom I love dearly and know means well, immediately said, "You probably shouldn't work out every day! It's good for you to take some time to recover." It bothered me because going to the gym was a wonderful part of my day, and I didn't want any doubt to creep in and take that from me. I understood that I had to be better at letting these moments of advice go.

Even though I've lost so much weight and have seen the results of committing to a plan, I still find it difficult to brush off opinions. Now, I don't need to lose another 100 pounds, but I'm still on my own plan and committing to new goals each day. I still watch my food intake, work out every day, and improving myself every way I can. I'm human, so sometimes I mess up and binge. If I think it's appropriate, I'll do a short diet or extra workout. No matter what, I'm doing my thing, and other people do not have the right to steer me in the wrong direction.

Once, my best friend pointed out that he thought the 1,500-calorie diet I had created for myself at the time was unhealthy. Even after losing 140 pounds, I still felt thrown off by my friend's opinion. We were hanging out, watching a movie, and I couldn't focus. I was so distracted that I spent the entire movie figuring out the macronutrients in my diet that day.

For those of you interested, macronutrients are the breakdown of the calories you consume. There are three categories: protein, carbs, and fat. Each calorie you consume has a percentage of all three. For people trying to lose large amounts of weight, macronutrients are less important than for a bodybuilder. It's more of an issue that comes into play when you are going from in-shape to athletic. Measuring macronutrients helps you go the extra distance, but they are pretty irrelevant when you are trying to shave off fifty pounds.

My point here is that I spent extra time calculating the nutritional value of my meals for the day. I discovered that my macros were split: 28 percent carbs, 38 percent fat, and 34 percent protein. That's pretty damn balanced for eating only 1,500 calories. I felt vindicated. I had been on the right track all along. Even though my friend knows a lot about fitness, his advice only distracted me from my goals.

84

Listening to other people's advice cost me time and emotional energy, and, oftentimes, veered me off my plan. Don't let other people's opinions do the same for you. I cannot stress this enough: *You* get to decide *your* path. If you want to take a day off, you can. If you want to work out every day, then go for it! If you want to go a full month without a cheat day, then just do it! Take your time finding out what you love about your weight loss. People will want to help you, and the best way they can do that is to support you. They can cheer you on for every pound lost and every lesson learned. This is a learning experience for you and those around you. They will see you bettering yourself, and they will want to stop giving advice and start taking direction. You made the decision to start this process for yourself and for them, but no matter what road you decide to take there will be opinions along the way. You have to brace yourself and keep your eyes on the end goal.

Justifications

The other type of bullshit you'll encounter is your own justifications: the way you rationalize skipping a workout, how you decide to take the night off of your food plan, or when you decide to let yourself slide. These are the times you let yourself down.

I see this all the time with people I train. It comes in big and small ways. People will justify shorter workout times, fewer miles to walk, or more calories than they'd planned. For example, I trained a woman who was on a plan that wasn't helping her lose weight. She'd been on it for a while—for some months. I gave her a new plan, and asked when she'd start the new plan. She responded, "I'll start Monday." It was Wednesday, and she'd start on Monday. To be clear, she was on a plan that she knew didn't work, but she's waiting to start an effective plan until Monday. We've all been there; I know I have. I can't count how many "I'll start tomorrows" I've said over the years in my life. You can't be your own reason for stopping.

> You've got to trust the plan. You've got to give yourself over to the process

You've got to trust the plan. You've got to give yourself over to the process. You've got to be all in, and you can't take shortcuts. Suffering through another five days of an ineffective plan is not going to help. Justifying your procrastination is not an option anymore, not when you want better for yourself.

Another justification for cheating or taking a break comes in the form of social pressure.

Friends will try to give you reasons to cheat on your plan to have fun with them. Again, this is common because your friends don't realize they're doing it. This time, instead of telling you what works (in terms of weight loss or a healthy life), they are encouraging you to believe that you can take a cheat day. They'll say, "We miss you!" or, "We haven't seen you in forever!" They'll say, "You look great—just come out with us! We'll only go to one bar."

You know it will never just be one bar or one drink; once

you're out, you want to enjoy yourself. Even if you are just going out for a casual lunch, chances are that you will be going to a place that serves pizza or Mexican food or something else equally unhealthy. These are potential weight gainers, PWGs.

During my first year of weight loss, I gave up a lot of ground by caving to peer pressure. Even though I was so dedicated to my workouts, I still let other people persuade me to break my routines. After a full work-week of treadmill and standing bike, I was willing to take any excuse to let down. I'd go out with my friends and binge. I'd gain back most of the weight I'd lost during the week. If it wasn't my friends, it was my family—they'd ask me to come over for dinner, and I'd give in, knowing

No one else is creating the life you want for you

that I'd be eating seconds and thirds. These people meant well; they wanted to see me and spend time with me, and they felt that I had been absent from their lives. But returning to my old habits was a choice that felt right for them, yet was not beneficial for me. They'd bring with them the temptation of going all out—or even just eating what I used to eat—and I was the one who suffered the consequences.

It's really easy to cave. You start telling yourself, "You know, I can afford a cheat day," or, "I don't need to work out today." Your friends and family love you, so they are going to baby you. But that babying will keep you stagnant! Of course, it is good for them if you skip out on your workout or come eat with them. It satisfies their needs for friendship and companionship (and justifies their own hamburger or what-ever). What they are not thinking of is what is good for you, and what is good for you is sticking to your plan!

Over time, those lies work themselves into your brain. It's a pattern I find happening over and over again. I'll get really motivated, I'll spend a week or two following my plan, and then I'll suddenly feel the temptation to blow it. I want to go out and get food—even though I know it will set me back. Now, cravings are normal. If I'm having a low-calorie day, I know I'm gonna crave chicken strips just as much as any other day. The feeling I'm referring to is not a normal craving. It is an emotional and physical craving—a lie that whispers that I am missing out on life because I am not eating junk food with my friends. In my head, I know the right move is to just suck it up and continue doing my thing and be healthy, but then I start to believe those whispers in my head: "I need to have a life. I look good enough right now. I can restart tomor-row." Sometimes I even use the excuse, "I need to go out for my mental health and just overall happiness." In my heart, though, I know that these are just excuses.

These small excuses are why losing weight takes so much time. They are the reason that losing my first seventy pounds took me so much longer than losing my second seventy pounds. Buckling down for three months makes a huge difference. You might even be able to reach your goals in that short amount of time. What often happens is that a person lasts two weeks and then takes a cheat day or two. Those cheat meals can set you back three to four days. Now you have to start the process over again. At this rate, with every month of effort you put in, you're only getting two and a half weeks' worth of results. These small backward steps will delay you so much. Trust me,

> Sometimes you have to change your surroundings in order to support yourself

I know you want to go out and have fun with your friends, but please just keep your head down and knock this out. It's going to suck, and it's going to take some time, but every decision you make deviating from your plan sets you back. My point is that it's okay to have something you are focused on, and sometimes that's going to occupy the free time you had before. You know what will benefit you in the long run. Stay focused and aim for that long-term goal. Stay positive—you know what you're doing!

I really want this to sink in. Let's look at an example. Say you want to lose thirty pounds. If you work out without interruptions, it will take you three months and three weeks to lose that much (with a calorie deficit of 1,000). If you stay on track every day except on Saturdays, it will take you four months and three weeks (same calories deficit). If you give up both days on the weekends, it will take you six months of nonsense to do something you could have done in three.

Now I know there are moments where you really feel like you need to go out and have fun. I still get those feelings when I need to lose weight, but, trust me, it's not worth it. Speaking from experience, if you go out, you might have an okay time, but you also just set yourself back. In three months of time, you can either be 100 percent done, or you can be halfway done! During the first year and a half of my workouts, I had so many setbacks. I routinely lost a lot of weight during the week and then binged, packing down six to seven thousand calories on the weekends. Those binges cost me so much in the long run. I wish I had known what kind of effect those days would have, and I wish I had taken up persistence early on. Instead, I let the bullshit of other people's excuses and lies become my own excuses.

This is attainable for you. It's not too big of a challenge

No one else is creating the life you want for you. The end deal is that it's your life. No one else is busting their ass for you except you. No one can tell you what's right because, chances are, they just don't know. Don't let the bullshit run your life, and don't let these messages get in your head. Your journey is your own.

I was just like you when I started this process. I wanted to lose the weight so badly that I would do almost anything to make it happen. I eventually did it, and all of this—the workouts, the failed diets, the wasted time, the extreme weight loss stretches, the binges, the criticism, the judgments—I certainly did it all for myself, but, just as importantly, I did it for you. I literally took my shovel and cleared the snow for miles to make a smooth path for you all. There is an easy way to lose weight and a hard way to lose weight. I started out by trying all the hard ways. You can pay the dumb tax and do it yourself, or I can show you such an easier way. Take the easy path!

CHAPTER EIGHT

Mindset

When your excitement wears off, you will hit a point of tiredness. You will just want to go back to your old habits. When weight loss gets tough, I want you to be able to push through the difficulty, keep your mental game strong, and hit the pavement when you feel like overanalyzing.

Priorities

In order to make this work, it has to be your number one priority. As I've shared, I tried to lose weight many times—and I failed. If I had to pinpoint one specific reason that I failed so many times before, I'd say it was because I did not have the discipline to put my health first. I let other aspects of my life take priority.

Losing weight is like any other goal in your life: it takes intentionality. If you want to be a more positive person, you have to make a conscious effort from the time you wake up to the time you go to bed to be positive. You have to practice over and over until it becomes part of you. It has to become second nature—and that takes repetition! Losing weight takes the same kind of concentration. I couldn't think about anything else. And, yeah, it did suck, but losing over 100 pounds is a big deal. It can't be a hobby. You can't just dabble in weight loss. In your head, you might think that it will be simple to chip off the pounds, week by week. But being casual about it is not going to work. You have to be all in. This is your main focus.

Some things are just not a priority. I ran out of Ziploc bags a week ago. I went to Target yesterday, and I forgot to pick some up. Will I get Ziploc bags? I don't know. Eventually, yeah. But it's not a priority. On the other hand, something which takes the same amount of effort—but is more important to me—of course I'll get that done. You can see this happen with anyone who has been a parent. I don't have kids at this point, but I imagine that after-school pickup is a pretty big interruption in a person's day: the kids can't drive themselves, so you have to stop what you're doing to pick them up. So what happens every day at 3:00 p.m.? Parents pick up their kids at school. Or if they don't personally pick them up, they figure out a way for the kid to be taken care of. And that's way harder than picking up plastic bags at Target! But that one gets done every day—no excuses—and the other gets put off for weeks. I have been to the store multiple times since I knew I was out of plastic bags, and I still haven't bought them. It's just not important to me. But parents make their kids a priority. Even if they have to leave work to go pick them up, they do. If they have to choose between their boss being pissed off and picking up their kids, they'll pick up their kids every single time. It's a priority.

That's the same mentality you have to have with weight loss. There will be times when you want to do other things. There will be times when you risk other people being upset. At the end of the day, weight loss stuff has to come first. Obviously, this level of dedication is easier for people who are in school—like I was at the time. But even with a full schedule and a family, you can make this a priority. You can still work a nine-to-five job and be thinking about losing weight all day. You can have a family and be thinking about it in the background. It just has to be the top priority in your life—almost all that you think about or talk about. The second you stop thinking about it, it's not a priority anymore. You just have to stay focused.

Let me give you an example of a time when I made an adjustment in my life to make space for my workouts. I travel for work a lot. With domestic travel, I have a routine I can fall back on, but this past year, I had an opportunity to travel internationally. I was going to Amsterdam. Now, everyone gains weight when they travel. It's just the way it is. This is especially true when you're in a place where you want to try the food and spend time seeing the sights. Finding a gym or a workout plan is simply low on the to-do list. I couldn't just cancel the trip, but I still wanted to prioritize my workouts. I knew I needed to make a plan.

The way I adjusted was to take vacation days after the work trip. When I came home, I joined my family on a trip to their beach house, and I focused on working out. I ate, slept, and exercised. That's all I did for an entire week, and it worked! I lost the weight I'd gained eating out and buying food while abroad. I was creative: Since I couldn't cancel the trip or make a way to work out sufficiently during the trip, I planned a post-trip vacation in which I only focused on getting my body right. Sometimes you have to change your surroundings in order to support yourself—in order to prioritize what you want to prioritize. Whatever you need to change to keep fitness as number one, change it. Let your surroundings support your weight loss.

There are only two directions: either forward or backwards. I can see this clearly throughout my weight loss journey. When I was complacent about where I was, I started to slide back. I'd go from losing two-and-a-half pounds a week, to losing a pound a week. Soon, I'd be losing no weight. Then I'd be gaining a half pound a week. Slowly, I went back to my pattern of gaining weight. You're either making progress, or you're going backwards. I don't know anyone who can stay the exact same weight forever.

There are only two directions: either forward or backwards

Even as a healthy person, most people gain and lose the same five to ten pounds. It's just what we do. It's almost harder to stay the same weight than it is to lose weight. You'd have to be very conscious of what you're doing every day to stay the same weight. Even drinking a glass of water changes that.

You're either gaining ground or losing it, and it's a snowball effect either way. When I lost thirty pounds, I was ecstatic and thought, "Wow. I can do this!" I saw I could do it and didn't want to lose momentum. I took that energy and ran with it. I didn't know what was going to happen; I just didn't want to lose my traction. I had come too far to go back. I was on the right path and took gaining weight off the table—it was no longer an option for me.

Master Your Mind—or It Masters You!

Part of losing weight is mastering your mind. Your mind can work for you, or it can work against you. When your mind works for you, it focuses on the tasks at hand and helps you move on to the next action step. Your mind can help you plan and strategize. When your mind works against you, it distracts you from your goals. It brings up worries and tempts you to waste time and energy.

For me, this struggle manifested in a strong temptation to obsess over details. I'd come to an aspect of weight loss that I did not fully understand, and I'd start worrying about it. For example, I'd ask myself, "What happens with my extra skin?" Or I'd realize that my family had a vacation planned and would worry about it, thinking, "Is it even possible to eat well on vacation? Should I cancel on them now? What will I do if I don't know what food options I'll have?" Even if that vacation was months down the road, I'd worry about it until it seemed like an insurmountable obstacle. With no immediate solution in sight, I'd feel overwhelmed. That feeling of being overwhelmed didn't always make me want to quit on the spot, but it did chip away at my motivation. When the worries and details piled up, I no longer wanted to give any effort. In this process, it is so easy to get caught in your head.

What I needed to do was wake up and realize that to-day's task was to push myself, eat like I was supposed to, and trust the process. Perhaps I needed to go to the grocery store to stock up on lunch food. Worrying about what I'd eat in two months distracted from what I had to do that day. Worrying about the physical process of weight loss just caused me to feel inadequate—even though those problems would take care of themselves! If you really tracked it, you would be surprised how many things we worry about that never actually happen or work themselves out on their own.

> *What I needed to do was wake up and realize that today's task was to push myself, eat like I was supposed to, and trust the process*

While it was tempting to get caught up in the small details, it was also easy to let big fears weigh me down. Not only would I be in my head about my vacation diet, I'd also let my mind run on about whether or not I could even accomplish what I started. I'd think, "You've never been able to lose weight before. Why do you think you can do it this time?" I'd hear the voice of self-criticism try to tear down my confidence, as I thought, "Why should anyone care what you think?" These thoughts were majorly destructive. They would discourage me from trying and put me in a negative mental space.

Eventually, I realized these thoughts were crazy, and I didn't have time for them. If I wanted to lose weight, I didn't have extra time or energy to worry about small details or about my personal fears. You don't have time for that shit either! Your own mind can be one of the biggest impediments to your own success. All of these worries, details, and questions live inside your head and distract you from actually accomplishing the work and might even cause you to give up on your dream! Every time you get discouraged with the minor details, it gets easier and easier to take days off or to give up completely. Don't let your mind distract you!

Stop overthinking your plan, your future, and the opinions of people around you

If you know me or have heard me speak, you know that one of my favorite pieces of advice is to stop overthinking. Stop overthinking your plan, your future, and the opinions of people around you. Stop analyzing and debating. I say it over and over again—to the point of annoyance—but I promise you that it is important advice. You have so much going on already. You have responsibilities, relationships, family obligations, and work or homework stressors. You don't need anything else on your plate.

Yes, I want you to make weight loss the most important part of your life. It is "the big rock" that goes in the jar first. It's the organizing principle. But that's different than stressing out about the small details. Prioritizing weight loss and holding the details lightly go hand in hand. You can be most successful at what's most important to you if it takes as little emotional and mental space as possible. This is why I stress routines, and this is why I created a simple system to track your progress. Whatever it takes for you to take action instead of overthinking your process—that's what you need to do. If you need to decide in advance what you're going to eat, then make a meal plan. If you need to eat the same food for breakfast each day to know how many calories you are taking in, then commit to the same breakfast every day. If you need to work out before going into the office, lay out your gym clothes the night before. Don't think about it! Just put on the clothes and go. Making decisions takes time and energy. Asking yourself what you're going to do next cracks the door open for your fears, worries, questions, and discouragement to come flooding in. Don't let your mind master you. Thinking about what will happen in the future, obsessing about what people think of you, or just longing for a break will not get you anywhere. Being in your head wastes your time and might even cause you to quit.

Instead, direct your focus on what matters. Your focus will guide your hours, days, and weeks. If you focus on all the small details, then you'll get tripped up on them. If you focus on the end goal, that's where you'll head. You can use focus along the way, too, to keep yourself positive and on track. It's pretty simple: If you focus on having a good day, then you will have a good day. If you focus on having a bad one—I can promise that your day will not go well. If you focus on not being able to eat the food you crave, then you will crave that food more. And, finally, if you focus on being a healthy you and bettering yourself, then that's where the world is going to take you.

Simply tell the universe what you want and receive it.

Just Try

Nothing moves us forward like action. Over and over again, we find that action is the remedy for our fears, problems, and pain. But—for whatever reason—there are so many times when we don't act! We get caught in our heads! We do not want to move forward because we are unsure of the future, and we are comfortable with our current habits. If you've been trying to lose weight, you know how true this is.

The best advice I can give you is to just do something. Try weight loss. Try my system. Try it, even just for an afternoon. Honestly, what will it cost you to try this? Maybe a few meals? An hour of walking or going to the gym? You can try out my system without much effort, and if you are not feeling it, then you can just as easily opt out. Try it for a day, a week, or a month. Anything you do will be improvement. What will not help your situation is thinking about it or making excuses. Try changing your patterns! Try eating less. Try incorporating exercise into your routine. Try keeping track of consumed and burned calories. Calculate your BMR. Nothing will change unless you take action.

I do not want you to waste your time, and I do not want you to stay overweight. I wrote this book to show you that you have the power to make big changes in your life. I lost

140 pounds, but I did it day by day, in small steps. This is attainable for you. It's not too big of a challenge. Focus on your points, focus on your routine, and get into a rhythm. It's your job to go through the motions, enjoy the process, and to not overthink it. If I could do it—while eating like a teenager and living in the real

Becoming emotionally and mentally healthy cannot happen quickly

world—so can you. Listen to your own advice and pursue your own goals. Find what works for you.

CHAPTER NINE

Holistic Health

Mental health is one of those topics people like to ignore. We like to focus on calories and moving down a shirt size and what food we can get away with eating. Those are tangibles. Mental health is difficult to handle because it's beneath the surface and touches on deeply rooted problems. As easy as it can be to ignore mental health, I've found it to be an important aspect of my weight loss journey.

Eventually, you'll have to ask yourself why you are overweight. A person does not become majorly overweight without having some kind of deeper problem to face. It might be an emotional, spiritual, or mental issue, but I can promise you it is not confined to the physical. Healthy people gain five, ten, even twenty pounds during different seasons of their life. If you are 320 pounds, like I was, your weight is a big sign that something else is going on.

I rejected the notion that mental health had anything to

Eventually, you'll have to ask yourself why you are overweight do with my weight for a long time. I used the classic excuse that I have bad genetics. I blamed my DNA for the way I looked and the way I lived. I wasn't wrong, either: I do have a genetic disposition toward obesity. What I wasn't willing to admit is that, while my genetics are an obstacle for me, genetics are only a small deterrent, not a major cause. I need to put in extra effort to stay healthy. Because of my genetics, I need to be careful about what I eat. Because of my genetics, I need to work out more regularly than other people. But my genetics do not automatically disqualify me from maintaining a healthy weight.

Say you are a healthy individual. Maybe you gain ten pounds on your honeymoon. Mental health is not causing that weight gain! You gained ten pounds in a scenario in which anyone would gain weight. These are times when programs like Weight Watchers become valuable. For people who are normally healthy, dieting and intensive workouts will be effective. Gaining thirty to fifty pounds, however, does not happen by accident.

As I've shared, I'm a binge eater. Even after I began losing weight, I held onto this habit. Because I wasn't willing (at first) to deal with my emotions, I kept repeating the same patterns. The truth was I wanted control. When I didn't get my way or when I was feeling bad about myself, I felt out of control, and I turned to the one aspect of my life in which I felt I had complete choice. Food put a smile on my face. Food made me feel better. I could choose to eat something that tasted good to me. Since I wasn't confident in myself and because I felt ashamed of myself, I looked to find comfort in something I could control. Some people turn to drugs or alcohol for the same reason. My vice has always been overeating.

Your personal struggle may be something completely different. I cannot speak to what you'll have to face, but from experience I can tell you that it's so important to deal with what's underneath the surface. That shit you're dealing with, all this stuff you don't want to address, is never going away on its own. If you don't let yourself feel and process your emotions all the way through, they are always going to be there. Sometimes you will feel your emotions more than other times, but I promise you they will come back if you don't tackle them head on. You genuinely need to let yourself process whatever feelings are there and deal with your life. Personally, I would rather have a meltdown for two weeks than suffer the consequences of suppressing my problems for the rest of my life. Looking inside of yourself is the only way to address the main issues in your life. I want to stress that they are not going away until you deal with them.

I believe in willpower—but only to a certain extent. If the rest of your life is in order, then willpower will be sufficient for you to lose weight. If you eat because you are unhappy or because you are self-conscious or because you want control in your life, willpower will only get you so far. You might be on track, motivated, and even see results of transformation, but—I am convinced—these results will not last. Eventually, you will return to the patterns that got you where you were in the first place. No matter how determined, you will only get so far without looking inside yourself. You have to deal with your feelings. You have to see them through—all the way.

Stress

Emotional problems follow us around because they are part of us. Sometimes, however, outside factors can affect our general health. Research shows that stress impacts our lives in many negative ways. I hate to break it to you, but body weight is one of those ways. I've had plenty of doctors tell me a stressed mind restricts a person's weight loss. The stress hormone, cortisol, makes you crave sweet and sugary foods. Sweet and sugary foods are a big category in PWGs (potential weight gainers). On top of craving sweet foods, over time, stress begins to restrict your body functions, including, some of the time, your ability to lose weight properly!

Stress is another demon in your life keeping you from the body you want

I really wish there was a way around this fact, but, for all of my wishing, it is still the reality we have to deal with. Honestly, I find it incredibly frustrating. Stress and weight gain build upon each other. I've already discussed the judgment and social ostracism overweight people experience. The emotional weight of those small experiences and the burden of shame make for a lot of stress! More stress makes it even harder for you to lose weight, which produces even more stress—you get the picture. It's a downward spiral.

Stress is another demon in your life keeping you from the body you want. I really encourage you to assess your life situation. What is causing you stress? Not all stressors are voluntary, but I bet you can take a few actions in your life to decrease the stress in your life. It could be as simple as shifting a morning routine. If you need to have that cup of coffee before you see anyone else, then make it a priority! Do you need a morning walk before work to clear your head? Do that! If you need to leave earlier to avoid stressful traffic, if you need to change your carpool to avoid a chatty Cathy, or if you need to say no to a weekend trip to save money, then do it. Your dreams are worth these adjustments. You need to focus on your goals, and that means giving up the little things that add stress to your life.

Decreasing stress could also mean making bigger changes. Do you need to find a new housing situation? Do you need a different position at work or a new job entirely? Are there relationships causing you stress? Do you need to set different boundaries or seek new friends? These are difficult changes. They will take courage, and they will take time. Believe me when I say your health is worth it. When the rest of those stresses go away, you will free yourself to work on what you want to work on. And, if you're reading this book, I know you've chosen a big goal—and a worthy one, which will make your life so, so much better. Losing weight is a lot of energy, time, and work—don't let stress make the process more difficult.

The truth is that you only have a limited amount of time

and energy in your life. Spend it on chasing goals that will actually bring you fulfillment. Status, money, and popularity will only bring so much change to your life. But emotional and physical health are priceless. Being confident in yourself and comfortable in your own body will change your life in huge ways. Let go of other stressors and focus in on what can bring you joy.

Five Ways I Reduce Stress

The Gym as a Place of Belonging

As I've said over and over, you've got to deal with what's on the inside. There's no better way to combat what's going on inside than to find a place where you can connect with people. A key element in my holistic health is actually my workout at the gym.

The gym has not always been a comfortable place for me. As an obese person, I felt intimidated by the gym. I felt embarrassed and out of place. I don't know if you'll ever feel completely comfortable in a gym, but I do know you'll be more successful if you have a dedicated time and space to work out and a place to connect with others. Contrary to popular misconception, the gym can be a place of belonging.

Losing weight does not have to be a lonely journey. Now, can you do at-home workouts and run/walk/hike outside? Yes, absolutely. Whatever works for you. Whatever helps you burn what you need to burn. If walking around the park is your thing, then that's great. Keep it up. My guess is that there will be cold and rainy days, and there will be times when working out at home won't be fun. The truth is that weather is no excuse to skip the workout.

Having guests staying in your basement (where you keep the treadmill) is no excuse. The gym is consistently available. It's a dedicated space for working out, it's filled with machines and tools to help you burn calories, and it's accessible to you most hours of the day.

But the gym's biggest asset to you is its community. I guarantee it.

As I've talked about, being overweight influences your mind. You start to believe that everyone will judge you. You'll believe it at the grocery store, and you'll believe it at the gym. There is a big misconception that people are judgmental at the gym. Big people think that, just like everywhere else, others won't want to be around you. And it's not just big people—everyone is worried about being judged at the gym.

But this just hasn't been my experience at all. I've been to hundreds of gyms in the Southwest, and I have never felt judged. Not in a single gym. People at the gym are focused on their own workouts and their own next steps. People are there because they are trying to grow themselves. They don't care that you're at a different level; they are excited for you to be there with them!

Going to work out is not an elite activity. It is not a club.

107

People respect that you are there for the same reason they are: to better yourself. Because of that, there's a sense of community that develops with the people you go to the gym with, even if you never speak with them. You might see someone outside the gym who works out with you, and there's a base sense of camaraderie. There have been times when I see someone wearing a shirt from a gym I go to, and suddenly I have something in common with a stranger. It's a shared experience.

Don't be scared to approach people and ask them questions! I used to think to myself, "I really don't know what I'm doing." Then I started asking people questions. I did when I was big, and I still ask people questions now that I'm fit. Ask what works for people (a motion or machine or routine), and people will help you! In fact, the gym is the one place I've seen people who are really in shape help other people for no reason. I've asked men and women for help and no one's ever been rude about a question I had. It doesn't matter if the other person is in better shape; as long as you ask politely, they're probably going to be helpful. People are honestly kind at the gym. You are all in it together.

Of course, there will be people who are more advanced than you at the gym. Definitely. There will also be people who you are further along than. But you have a choice here. You can choose to be intimidated, or you can choose to be inspired. I don't know about you, but when I look at someone who is just killing it at the gym, I'm impressed! And I feel motivated! Being around successful people inspires me. When you're at the gym, you will have the opportunity to be around people who model your own trajectory. Try to be around these people. Watch their gym routines, if you can. You will not be able to do what they're doing right away, but seeing them will help you imagine where you're going. This is different than comparing yourself to others. You are still only competing with yourself, and you use other people's work ethic and results as inspiration.

It is difficult for anyone to imagine a new future for themselves. As I've reiterated, I grew up as an overweight kid. I'd never known what it would be like to be an average weight. Because I didn't know what I was aiming for, there were a few times when I seriously considered stopping my weight loss process. At 270 pounds, having lost fifty pounds, I felt amazing. I looked at myself in the mirror and hardly recognized who I had become. I had jumped down several sizes, bought new clothes, and felt like a new man. I congratulated myself and thought, "I could stay at 270 forever. I'm good." After a couple weeks of complacency, I started to see that at 270 I was still way overweight. I looked at what other people accomplished, and I was inspired to do better. I hopped back on my routine, and I lost another thirty pounds. At 240 pounds, I looked at myself in the mirror and congratulated myself. I was the lightest I had been in years. I looked good. I was healthier than ever before. I felt I could live at 240 forever. A few weeks later, I leveled with myself again: I still had weight to lose if I wanted to be healthy. At each twenty-pound mark after that point, I questioned whether I should stop. Each time, what motivated me to continue was seeing other people (at the gym) who had worked to be at a better place. Watching them, I saw where I wanted to be, and I started to believe I could get there.

Being around them not only gave me the chance to watch and learn, I could also talk with them! For me, the gym was a community of acceptance and growth: I learned to take advantage of the experience in the room. The people around me knew how to do different exercises, they knew effective ways to burn calories, and they had tactics for growing more muscle. It was like having free coaches around all the time. If you get to know these people, they will also help you make adjustments and find your best routine.

The gym community will give you confidence and a sense of belonging and also help you learn how to exercise a little better. These people have your back!

The Gym as a Place of Mental Health

Certainly, the gym is a place to work on our bodies. But it's also a place to work on our minds. I discovered this simply by bringing my phone with me to the gym.

Having a phone does a couple of things for you: one, watching a show or listening to music helps the time go by. Cardio isn't fun for everyone. I know I had my struggle with getting excited about it. There's no way anyone can go ninety minutes on a machine and not feel bored. It's impossible. I know I needed distraction. I was logging long hours! Especially at first, I'd be at the gym all day, but with my phone it didn't feel like torture. Honestly, I would jump on the bike, pull out my iPad, and watch music videos or Netflix shows. When I first started working out, I was really into The Office, and I'd binge-watch entire seasons during my workouts. I would watch entire movies at the treadmill. Even now, while I am in way better shape than I was when I started, I still need something to make cardio go by faster. YouTube videos, movies, and TV shows help the time pass.

But more importantly, watching a show or listening to a podcast teaches you something! You're not only improving your body, you're also improving your mind. And, honestly, I love that people make content—whether it's a podcast or a YouTube series or something else—about their passions. It's fascinating to learn from someone who's passionate. And it feels so good to learn something new! Even when I do my normal workout without consuming any content, I feel good about myself—like I've done what I needed to do. But when I learn something new while working out, I feel genius status. I feel on top of the world. I'm learning things, improving my body, and kicking ass at life. It's next level.

Plus, if you have specific questions about how to work out, what to eat, or how to use a particular machine, YouTube has the answer. I use YouTube as a resource for all kinds of questions. There are plenty of videos teaching you the right form and giving you new ideas. If there is an exercise I want to learn to do, there are plenty of videos to show me how. Recently, I looked up a front squat. It works the front of your legs instead of the back of your legs, and it's not something I'm very good at. It's also hard because it works your wrists.

If you don't do it right, not only do you miss the benefits of the workout, you might also really hurt yourself. The videos I found showed me what to do and warned me about common mistakes. It was only about ten minutes of content, and I watched it while I was on the bike—which means I wasted no time, since I was going to do time on the bike anyway. Then, as I tried the squat, I literally put the phone on the floor next to me as I tried it out. Educating myself gave me confidence to try something new!

Watching them, I saw where I wanted to be, and I started to believe I could get there

You can also look up entertainment training videos: these are from media personalities. While these shows focus on comedy, they often have small bits of helpful information. I've used their tips in my personal workouts and as I'm training other people.

Gym culture may seem overwhelming. But I promise you that the gym can be an encouraging and educational space. Burning calories on the treadmill is amazing, but transforming your mind at the same time, with podcasts and other educational material, doubles the benefit you're receiving. It's all connected: your mind, your body, your well-being.

Taking it Slow

The good news is that you don't have to deal with all of your problems at once. Pacing yourself is important. You don't have to sit in a room and fix yourself in an afternoon. In fact, you can't. Becoming emotionally and mentally healthy cannot happen quickly. Just take it day by day. Take small, conscious steps (like joining a gym community or starting a podcast) to better yourself mentally and emotionally, and those small steps will add up. For me, the biggest hurdle was simply realizing that my binge eating was more than just a physical problem. I asked myself why I was eating so much. Slowly, it dawned on me that my emotional issues were not confined to mealtimes. I noticed that my confidence was low throughout the day, whether or not food was involved. I connected my insecurity with the times I would ask for other people's validation, withhold my own opinion, or follow another's lead. I couldn't fix all of these habits in one day, but I slowly began to change. A couple of times a week, I'd stop myself from asking people where to go for lunch or what to do on my day off. I didn't need anyone's validation. I began to trust myself and make my own decisions.

It was an amazing process because this change was not an outward one, but it really made a difference. Confidence became easier as I focused on it; in a sense, our growth follows our focus. This is natural to all kinds of positive growth. If someone tells you that you are funny, you'll start telling more jokes, and then you'll get better at comedy. I felt rewarded for my confidence and, consequently, felt even more confident. I

our growth follows our focus

found myself in a positive cycle. My awareness led to changes which led to positive results which led to more confidence.

I'm not sure if this is true for everyone, but when I start a new project, I get really excited. I go all in, and it's all I can think about. I set out an ambitious plan for today, for the next few weeks, and for the year. I'll give the new endeavor 100 percent of my focus. And I am successful—for a couple of weeks. Then I start to lose steam. I've done this with weight loss programs, with school work, and with business ideas. I go hard, and then I get distracted. I'm not saying that you shouldn't get excited. Being excited is great. You should be excited about your weight loss journey. I just also want you to remember that you will experience fluctuation in your feelings during this process. The lows can be really discouraging. Taking the process day by day helps manage the rollercoaster of emotions. You don't have to do it all at once: today has manageable, concrete steps. Focus on those small steps. Do it a little at a time. You don't have to tackle it all in a single day.

Losing weight is always more than a number on a scale

You can't lose the weight and become emotionally healthy all in one week. This journey requires patience and con-sistency. It is important to keep making little strides.

Losing weight is always more than a number on a scale. The process involves your whole self. Motivation alone will not fix you. You need to be okay with yourself emotionally. This is what weight loss programs and reality TV shows miss. While they might work on paper, they do not address your personal issues and, consequently, will not last.

If what you're currently doing is easy, it's not growth. Growth is difficult. Growth can be painful. If you wanted to do what you need to do, you'd already be there. Growth means facing what we do not want to do. Fortunately, pushing through the discomfort has great rewards. Compared to a life burdened by stress, emotional problems, and physical weight, a healthy body, heart, and mind make life a cakewalk. Trust me. You don't want to miss out.

CHAPTER TEN

Life After

For me, there are two time periods in my life: life before my weight loss and life after my weight loss. I cannot emphasize how drastically different these two lives were for me. The difference between normal people and celebrities—that's the difference between my obese life and my fit life.

If you're wondering if all this work will be worth it, I'm here to tell you that it's the best thing that could ever happen.

You Don't Know What You Don't Know

It's been about five years now since I've been overweight, and I still forget what I look like sometimes. I'll walk into my bathroom in the morning and be sincerely shocked to see someone who is not obese. I've lived the majority of my life as the overweight guy. It was a part of my identity for a long time to have extra weight on me. To not live that life anymore still blows my mind. I really don't know if that surprise ever goes away. Fortunately, it's not a bad feeling. The feeling is actually a nice reminder of all the hard work I've put in and how far I've come since day one.

It reminds me of when I graduated high school. I went through the graduation ceremony, celebrating and feeling excited about the future. I woke up the next day, and that's when it all hit me. I had put my head down and worked for four years, and then I achieved my goal. It didn't feel real. Part of the strangeness of graduation was also that I could never have my high school experience again. The organizing features of my life had shifted. My schedule would never be the same. My friends would go in different directions. I wouldn't see my teachers every day. I would have to find new pursuits and new goals. It was difficult for me to wrap my head around what my new life would look like. I had only known school. The same goes for a life without extra weight. Before I achieved my weight loss goals, I honestly did not know what it could be like to experience life as a healthy person.

Before I achieved my weight loss goals, I honestly did not know what it could be like to experience life as a healthy person

How could I? It's simply true that you don't know what you don't know.

I like to demonstrate this concept by thinking of it in terms of income. Imagine if everyone in the world made $40K a year. What if people never experienced luxurious times or ate expensive foods, and if everyone lived on basic items. If no one knew any other way to live, then everyone would be content! We'd all feel completely comfortable in our lifestyle, and rightfully so. We could pay for food, avoid or pay off debt, and afford solid cars and homes. We would simply have no clue how it feels to make more money. Expensive vacations, luxurious dinners, new cars, and remodeled houses would not be options for anyone, and no one would think to want them. We would not know what money could do to change our experience. Being severely out of shape creates a similar situation. I felt fine where I was at and had a good life. I had fulfilling friendships and hobbies, and I was successful in school. But I could not imagine what life could look like at another level.

Now that I've arrived, I'm asking you to believe me. It's another level.

The Better Life

Life gets better as you become healthier! In a few months from now, your life will be completely different. You'll notice a change in your mood and in your attitude facing new challenges. You'll have started a wonderful new chapter, and I promise you, you'll wish you would have done this sooner. Let me share with you a few of the ways my life improved as I lost weight.

What I first noticed was the difference in the way the general public treats me. I'd grown used to glances and how those around would ignore me. My confidence is what has made me feel the biggest difference: I'm not afraid anymore. I approach everything with a positive mindset and the results have really taken me by surprise. When I become a regular at a place (my gym, the local Target, the smoothie place down the street, even Cane's), the staff remembers me and starts talking to me when I walk in. People on the street open doors for me. It's strange, but people are just kind.

When I first posted pictures of my new self, people from my past started popping out of the woodwork. People I didn't even remember meeting would text or message me on social media to tell me how good I looked and how proud they were of me. Certainly, I had the support of my close family and friends, but other people—people I hardly knew—supported me too.

Without the extra weight, I can tell that other people find me more approachable—I don't put up a wall anymore. It's not me vs. the world any longer. I slip into my old mentality sometimes and think, "Why would someone want to be my friend?" But I quickly shake it off. Why wouldn't they? I am someone who showed that you don't have to let the world decide who you are. I stopped allowing my size to also label my personality. The Aaron who's here is worth getting to know.

I can't tell you how many times people failed to show me kindness when I was overweight. I didn't feel slighted that strangers didn't approach me—that was normal for me. Now my normal has changed; that lack of kindness and empathy is gone. People, instead, compliment me on my clothes and hair. People will come up to me in a store or at the gym and strike up a conversation—something they never used to do, but, then again, I never used to care about myself enough to put in this effort. When you care about yourself, it shows, and I was finally at a place where I could show my personality through my style. The other day, I was at a bar, and after chatting with the bartender he offered me a drink on the house. Just because. Just to be nice. Just because we were chatting. As a pay-it-forward moment. This kind of everyday kindness still blows my mind. Do people live like this all the time? It's sad to say, but something like that would never have happened to me when I was overweight. Why? Because I let my negative feelings toward myself and those around me overshadow my best aspects. Now that I was confident and comfortable in my own skin, I could finally be able to share myself with the world.

Losing weight will change your life for the better, so much more than an extra slice of pizza on a Saturday night.

As you lose weight, you'll have the positive reinforcement from your close friends and close family members. But you will also start to interact with wider circles. You are going to have so many friends, and so many new people are going to get to know you. It'll be a completely new life, one you're excited to share. Who is this newly excited and attractive person? That attractive person is YOU! You get to live that life because you are enough, and you deserve it.

As I saw my own improvement, I started to take pride in myself. As I treated myself well, I started to hold my head a little higher as I walked. When you are happy with yourself physically and mentally, it just changes everything. You will feel better about your own decisions and opinions.

My confidence has been the biggest game-changer, but I have also benefited from other shifts. Before I lost weight, I never enjoyed sports. If my friends went to play football, I didn't join them. It didn't sound fun. Even active leisure activities like hiking were simply not options for me. Walking up a mountain might be enjoyable for healthy people, but imagine walking up a hill with a 200-pound backpack! No thank you! It was just not fun.

Now, I'm excited for a challenging hiking expedition. I have the ability and confidence to try new sports. If you had told 320-pound Aaron that he would, in the future, try and enjoy skiing, he would have laughed in your face. I also enjoy healthy foods, and I don't like some of the unhealthy foods I used to eat. My body has adjusted to better habits, and I enjoy foods that nourish my body. There are still some vegetables I stay away from (I don't think I'll ever learn to like carrots), but I have learned to like other vegetables. My pallet has expanded from that of a child, and I enjoy more food.

As far as my daily habits, even now that I'm healthy, I still follow my plan. I'm not trying to lose fifty pounds, but I still want to monitor my food intake, exercise every day, and set goals for myself. The difference is that I enjoy my lifestyle. I look forward to the gym and to taking care of myself because I see the difference it has made in my life.

Your life is about to get so much better, and you have yourself to thank! I'm so damn happy for you. I'm excited for you to get started and find the foods you like and don't like. I'm excited for you to find a new hobby through exercise. Maybe it will be a league sport, or maybe you will reconnect with friends through hiking. You might even make new friends at the gym! I can't wait for you to lose your first ten pounds and have the feeling of "I can actually do this" for the first time. I'm ecstatic for you to lose more weight and get new clothes. I'm elated for you to actually go shopping where you like and have the clothes that fit. I'm overjoyed for you to no longer label yourself as "the fat person," and for others to see you for more than just your weight. And, finally, I'm thrilled for you to take this journey to find who you are.

Your life is about to get so much better, and you have yourself to thank!

The Invitation

t's really important to know who is going to help you in this process: who will be on your team.

When I made the decision to lose weight, I didn't tell anyone—not even my family or closest friends. In all the times I had tried to lose weight before, I had never lost more than twenty pounds. I wasn't ready to admit to anyone what I was trying to do until I had reached that twenty-pound mark.

Eventually, I started to lean on my friends who were body-builders or were in nutrition classes. When I had questions, I felt comfortable asking them, knowing they had training I could learn from and that they wanted the best for me. As I spent more time at the gym, I developed relationships there. My gym friends understood my priorities and supported me in my decisions. I learned how to use the machines at the gym and how to work out large, calorie-burning muscle groups. I learned about macronutrients and micronutrients and how to get what I needed while still eating an appropriate amount. These people became part of my team.

It's equally as important to know who is not on your team. I also learned to say no when friends wanted me to break my routines. I learned to lean on people who could help me and ignore those who tried to push me away from my goals. You can't expect everyone to understand what you are doing. In fact, most people will just not get it. I can guarantee you will feel alone in this process. I wish it weren't true, but it is. You are doing what is best for you, and other people might not get on board. Certainly, I had a base of friends cheering me on. At about the thirty-pound mark, people who had known me for a long time began to notice my weight loss. They'd congratulate me. At about the fifty-pound mark, acquaintances and classmates who hadn't seen me in a while began noticing and commenting. My family was, of course, supportive. Even so, none of these people understood. They still wanted me to hang out with them, suggested I skip the gym, or tried to give me excuses to eat extra calories. But these little excuses only held me back. I learned that I needed to put myself first and separate myself from people who discouraged me.

All of this is coming, and I want you to be prepared. As much as possible, surround yourself with people who will help you get to where you need to be. It doesn't have to be many people. It could just be a few key individuals. Having people who understand what you're doing and why you're doing it will be a source of great energy for you in the difficult and discouraging times of your weight loss journey. You need people building you up and teaching you how to be effective.

Knowing what I know now, after all that weight loss, I

can't believe what I was doing when I started. The way I began looks nothing like my current routines. I had no idea what I was doing. Absolutely none. I spent a lot of time doing exercises that weren't actually beneficial. I wasted a lot of calories on foods that are popularly thought of as healthy even though they actually aren't. I also listened to the wrong people—to the friends who were offering the easy way out and encouraging me to give up. Part of the reason I share my story with you is so you can have a support system from the beginning. I want to save you the dumb tax—and save you real dollars as well. Personal trainers are expensive! Starting at a young age, I'd had different personal trainers. For about a month or two, I'd utilize them. Personal trainers are $40-$60 for a half hour. You know how many half hours you will be spending in the gym? That's a lot of money. I couldn't afford that, and my guess is you can't afford it either.

That's why I want to provide something different. I want to help you. If you show up with a reason to change your life (and I hope this book has given you one), then I'll come with an action plan. I can be a consultant and guide for you—I'll tell you what to eat and how to exercise. I'll help you make a manageable plan—one that works specifically for you. I don't want you to make the same mistakes I did. I don't want you to have to waste your sweat trying to learn a million different things. I want to get you the information and help you in timely ways, so you can make the most of your workouts, mealtimes, and pocketbook.

You don't have to do this alone. I know what you are

facing and where you are headed. I want you to reach your goals! Losing weight will change your life for the better, so much more than an extra slice of pizza on a Saturday night. I understand that losing weight is an emotional, mental, and physical journey. Let me be your guide.

This is my story. I've shared with you my life—all the vulnerable and challenging moments, what caused me to change, and how I lost 140 pounds—with hopes of helping you. If you have someone who's helping you already, that's great. Do what works. Keep it up. I am totally stoked for you. But if you're looking for a place to start or to change your current routine, then this book is the sign you've been waiting for.

Even if you're not looking for a consultant or coach, please reach out! It's one of the biggest privileges of my life to meet people who are, or who have been, overweight and who want to work towards health. Because I've been there too, we get each other in ways other people do not understand. I'm on all the social media platforms—absolutely reach out and share with me your story! I love to connect with anyone and everyone, no matter where they are on their weight loss journey. Whether it's one pound or one hundred, the minute you decide to put yourself first, you will start to see results. I want to be the first to celebrate with you because you deserve it! I'm a real person just like you, and my quality of life has changed dramatically through weight loss. I've learned how to improve myself and enjoy the process. I've learned that it's worth taking care of myself. It's a huge learning curve and a big adventure. I'm inviting you along. Wherever you are in the journey, I'm asking you to take your next steps and genuinely hope you say yes.

You're here, reading this right now, for a reason. You deserve the best kind of change you could possibly make for yourself. I'm so stoked for you and your journey.

Now, let's get started!

Aaron's Most Common Foods

Tracking your calories is going to help you significantly in this weight loss journey. I know it helped me. But at first, it's going to feel overwhelming. It's a lot to look up every item of food you want to eat and calculate its value.

I don't want you to be discouraged. It does get easier. As you practice, the process will soon be second nature to you, and you'll even start to remember some of your common meals. Today, I know the caloric value of most of the foods I regularly eat.

Making a list of your favorite foods is a helpful first step. To give you an example and some base knowledge, I've listed some of my favorite foods. You'll notice some lean toward the healthy side, while some definitely don't—and they are in no particular order. We're about balance and eating what makes us happy, and, as long as we keep track of it, we're doing great. So here it is! I encourage you to make a list of your own!

- Kodiak protein pancakes: 190 calories per serving
- Eggs: 70 calories each

- Frosted Mini Wheats: 210 per serving
- Quest bars: roughly 190 each
- Sarah Lee bread: 45 calories per slice
- Peanut butter: 2 Tbsp for 190
- Honey: 70 calories per Tbsp
- Justin's dark chocolate peanut butter cups: 210 per package
- Mini Hershey's, Special Dark: 136 for four pieces
- Chipotle: guac: 230 a serving; chicken: 180 per serving; cheese: 110 per serving; black beans: 120 per serving; sour cream: 110 per serving; tortilla: 300 each; white rice: 130 per serving
- Raising Cane's: chicken finger: 140 each; Cane's sauce: 173 each; fries: 291 per serving; toast: 120
- Frosted Flakes: 110 per serving
- Spicy shrimp avocado roll at Whole Foods: 380 per container
- Grapes: 62 calories per cup
- Strawberries: 49 calories per cup
- Cantaloupe: 54 calories per cup
- Eggos, buttermilk: 95 calories each
- Sirloin steak: 60 calories per ounce
- Cheese: roughly 100 calories per slice
- 85% lean ground beef: 60 calories per ounce
- Chick-fil-A: sandwich, 440 calories; nuggets, 34 calories each

- Pizza: Costco combo pizza, 1 slice: 680 calories; Sbarro's, cheese, 1 slice: 430 calories; general slice of pizza, cheese, 300 calories
- One cup of apples: 57 calories
- One cup of carrots: 53 calories
- Halo Top ice cream: 280–360 for an entire container
- Birds Eye Veggie Made cauliflower fries: 140 per serving
- Greek yogurt: 130 calories per serving
- Shrimp, seven medium, 85 calories
- Jimmy Johns: Turkey Tom, 510 calories; Club Lulu, 720 calories; BLT, 560 calories
- Potato chips, general: 150 calories per serving
- Deli meats (1 oz.): turkey, 25 calories; Buffalo chicken, 35 calories; pepperoni, 80 calories; salami, 110 calories

Now it's your turn! Make a list of your favorite foods, then look up the calories per serving and enter them here.

Your Favorite Foods

Food   Calories per Serving

_____   _____

_____   _____

_____   _____

_____   _____

_____   _____

_____   _____

_____   _____

_____   _____

_____   _____

_____   _____

_____   _____

Food   Calories per Serving

_____   _____

_____   _____

_____   _____

_____   _____

_____   _____

_____   _____

_____   _____

_____   _____

_____   _____

_____   _____

_____   _____

_____   _____

_____   _____

_____   _____

_____   _____

_____   _____

_____   _____

Journaling Pages

If you've looked up all of your favorite foods and entered the calorie count for each, you are ready to start losing weight the *Calories In Calories Out* way! You now know you need to keep track of what you eat and how many calories you burn during exercise. Great! To give you a head start, I've provided journaling pages you can use for the first few weeks. I encourage you to find a notebook, journal, or app that works for you and, most importantly, that you will actually *use*.

There is really no magic here. It's all about burning more calories than you take in. Let's get started!

Calories In:

Food   Total Calories

_____   _____

_____   _____

_____   _____

_____   _____

_____   _____

_____   _____

_____   _____

_____   _____

_____   _____

_____   _____

_____   _____

_____   _____

_____   _____

Calories Out:

Activity   Calories Burned

_____   _____

_____   _____

_____   _____

BMR: _____ Weight: _____ Date: _____

Calories In:

Food   Total Calories

_____   _____

_____   _____

_____   _____

_____   _____

_____   _____

_____   _____

_____   _____

_____   _____

_____   _____

_____   _____

_____   _____

_____   _____

Calories Out:

Activity   Calories Burned

_____   _____

_____   _____

_____   _____

BMR: _____ Weight: _____ Date: _____

Calories In:

Food   Total Calories

_____   _____

_____   _____

_____   _____

_____   _____

_____   _____

_____   _____

_____   _____

_____   _____

_____   _____

_____   _____

_____   _____

_____   _____

Calories Out:

Activity   Calories Burned

_____   _____

_____   _____

_____   _____

BMR: _____ Weight: _____ Date: _____

Calories In:

Food   Total Calories

_____   _____

_____   _____

_____   _____

_____   _____

_____   _____

_____   _____

_____   _____

_____   _____

_____   _____

_____   _____

_____   _____

_____   _____

Calories Out:

Activity   Calories Burned

_____   _____

_____   _____

_____   _____

BMR: _____ Weight: _____ Date: _____

Calories In:

Food   Total Calories

_____   _____

_____   _____

_____   _____

_____   _____

_____   _____

_____   _____

_____   _____

_____   _____

_____   _____

_____   _____

_____   _____

_____   _____

Calories Out:

Activity   Calories Burned

_____   _____

_____   _____

_____   _____

BMR: _____ Weight: _____ Date: _____

Calories In:

Food   Total Calories

_____   _____

_____   _____

_____   _____

_____   _____

_____   _____

_____   _____

_____   _____

_____   _____

_____   _____

_____   _____

_____   _____

_____   _____

Calories Out:

Activity   Calories Burned

_____   _____

_____   _____

_____   _____

BMR: _____ Weight: _____ Date: _____

Calories In:

Food   Total Calories

_____   _____

_____   _____

_____   _____

_____   _____

_____   _____

_____   _____

_____   _____

_____   _____

_____   _____

_____   _____

_____   _____

_____   _____

Calories Out:

Activity   Calories Burned

_____   _____

_____   _____

_____   _____

BMR: _____ Weight: _____ Date: _____

Calories In:

Food   Total Calories

_____   _____

_____   _____

_____   _____

_____   _____

_____   _____

_____   _____

_____   _____

_____   _____

_____   _____

_____   _____

_____   _____

_____   _____

Calories Out:

Activity   Calories Burned

_____   _____

_____   _____

_____   _____

BMR: _____ Weight: _____ Date: _____

Calories In:

Food   Total Calories

_____   _____

_____   _____

_____   _____

_____   _____

_____   _____

_____   _____

_____   _____

_____   _____

_____   _____

_____   _____

_____   _____

_____   _____

Calories Out:

Activity   Calories Burned

_____   _____

_____   _____

_____   _____

BMR: _____ Weight: _____ Date: _____

Calories In:

Food   Total Calories

_____   _____

_____   _____

_____   _____

_____   _____

_____   _____

_____   _____

_____   _____

_____   _____

_____   _____

_____   _____

_____   _____

_____   _____

Calories Out:

Activity   Calories Burned

_____   _____

_____   _____

_____   _____

BMR: _____ Weight: _____ Date: _____

Calories In:

Food   Total Calories

_____   _____

_____   _____

_____   _____

_____   _____

_____   _____

_____   _____

_____   _____

_____   _____

_____   _____

_____   _____

_____   _____

_____   _____

Calories Out:

Activity   Calories Burned

_____   _____

_____   _____

_____   _____

BMR: _____ Weight: _____ Date: _____

Calories In:

Food   Total Calories

_____   _____

_____   _____

_____   _____

_____   _____

_____   _____

_____   _____

_____   _____

_____   _____

_____   _____

_____   _____

_____   _____

_____   _____

_____   _____

Calories Out:

Activity   Calories Burned

_____   _____

_____   _____

_____   _____

BMR: _____ Weight: _____ Date: _____

Calories In:

Food   Total Calories

_____   _____

_____   _____

_____   _____

_____   _____

_____   _____

_____   _____

_____   _____

_____   _____

_____   _____

_____   _____

_____   _____

_____   _____

Calories Out:

Activity   Calories Burned

_____   _____

_____   _____

_____   _____

BMR: _____ Weight: _____ Date: _____

Calories In:

Food   Total Calories

_____   _____

_____   _____

_____   _____

_____   _____

_____   _____

_____   _____

_____   _____

_____   _____

_____   _____

_____   _____

_____   _____

_____   _____

Calories Out:

Activity   Calories Burned

_____   _____

_____   _____

_____   _____

BMR: _____ Weight: _____ Date: _____

Calories In:

Food   Total Calories

_____   _____

_____   _____

_____   _____

_____   _____

_____   _____

_____   _____

_____   _____

_____   _____

_____   _____

_____   _____

_____   _____

_____   _____

Calories Out:

Activity   Calories Burned

_____   _____

_____   _____

_____   _____

BMR: _____ Weight: _____ Date: _____

Calories In:

Food   Total Calories

_____   _____

_____   _____

_____   _____

_____   _____

_____   _____

_____   _____

_____   _____

_____   _____

_____   _____

_____   _____

_____   _____

_____   _____

Calories Out:

Activity   Calories Burned

_____   _____

_____   _____

_____   _____

BMR: _____ Weight: _____ Date: _____

Calories In:

Food   Total Calories

_____   _____

_____   _____

_____   _____

_____   _____

_____   _____

_____   _____

_____   _____

_____   _____

_____   _____

_____   _____

_____   _____

_____   _____

Calories Out:

Activity   Calories Burned

_____   _____

_____   _____

_____   _____

BMR: _____ Weight: _____ Date: _____

Calories In:

Food   Total Calories

_____   _____

_____   _____

_____   _____

_____   _____

_____   _____

_____   _____

_____   _____

_____   _____

_____   _____

_____   _____

_____   _____

_____   _____

_____   _____

Calories Out:

Activity   Calories Burned

_____   _____

_____   _____

_____   _____

BMR: _____ Weight: _____ Date: _____

Calories In:

Food   Total Calories

_____   _____

_____   _____

_____   _____

_____   _____

_____   _____

_____   _____

_____   _____

_____   _____

_____   _____

_____   _____

_____   _____

Calories Out:

Activity   Calories Burned

_____   _____

_____   _____

_____   _____

BMR: _____ Weight: _____ Date: _____

Calories In:

Food   Total Calories

_____   _____

_____   _____

_____   _____

_____   _____

_____   _____

_____   _____

_____   _____

_____   _____

_____   _____

_____   _____

_____   _____

Calories Out:

Activity   Calories Burned

_____   _____

_____   _____

_____   _____

BMR: _____ Weight: _____ Date: _____

Calories In:

Food   Total Calories

_____   _____

_____   _____

_____   _____

_____   _____

_____   _____

_____   _____

_____   _____

_____   _____

_____   _____

_____   _____

_____   _____

_____   _____

Calories Out:

Activity   Calories Burned

_____   _____

_____   _____

_____   _____

BMR: _____ Weight: _____ Date: _____

Calories In:

Food   Total Calories

_____   _____

_____   _____

_____   _____

_____   _____

_____   _____

_____   _____

_____   _____

_____   _____

_____   _____

_____   _____

_____   _____

_____   _____

Calories Out:

Activity   Calories Burned

_____   _____

_____   _____

_____   _____

BMR: _____ Weight: _____ Date: _____

Calories In:

Food   Total Calories

_____   _____

_____   _____

_____   _____

_____   _____

_____   _____

_____   _____

_____   _____

_____   _____

_____   _____

_____   _____

_____   _____

_____   _____

Calories Out:

Activity   Calories Burned

_____   _____

_____   _____

_____   _____

BMR: _____ Weight: _____ Date: _____

Calories In:

Food   Total Calories

_____   _____

_____   _____

_____   _____

_____   _____

_____   _____

_____   _____

_____   _____

_____   _____

_____   _____

_____   _____

_____   _____

_____   _____

Calories Out:

Activity   Calories Burned

_____   _____

_____   _____

_____   _____

BMR: _____ Weight: _____ Date: _____

Calories In:

Food   Total Calories

_____   _____

_____   _____

_____   _____

_____   _____

_____   _____

_____   _____

_____   _____

_____   _____

_____   _____

_____   _____

_____   _____

_____   _____

Calories Out:

Activity   Calories Burned

_____   _____

_____   _____

_____   _____

BMR: _____ Weight: _____ Date: _____

Calories In:

Food   Total Calories

_____   _____

_____   _____

_____   _____

_____   _____

_____   _____

_____   _____

_____   _____

_____   _____

_____   _____

_____   _____

_____   _____

_____   _____

Calories Out:

Activity   Calories Burned

_____   _____

_____   _____

_____   _____

BMR: _____ Weight: _____ Date: _____

Calories In:

Food   Total Calories

_____   _____

_____   _____

_____   _____

_____   _____

_____   _____

_____   _____

_____   _____

_____   _____

_____   _____

_____   _____

_____   _____

_____   _____

Calories Out:

Activity   Calories Burned

_____   _____

_____   _____

_____   _____

BMR: _____ Weight: _____ Date: _____

Calories In:

Food   Total Calories

_____   _____

_____   _____

_____   _____

_____   _____

_____   _____

_____   _____

_____   _____

_____   _____

_____   _____

_____   _____

_____   _____

_____   _____

_____   _____

Calories Out:

Activity   Calories Burned

_____   _____

_____   _____

_____   _____

BMR: _____ Weight: _____ Date: _____

Calories In:

Food   Total Calories

_____   _____

_____   _____

_____   _____

_____   _____

_____   _____

_____   _____

_____   _____

_____   _____

_____   _____

_____   _____

_____   _____

_____   _____

Calories Out:

Activity   Calories Burned

_____   _____

_____   _____

_____   _____

BMR: _____ Weight: _____ Date: _____

Calories In:

Food   Total Calories

_____   _____

_____   _____

_____   _____

_____   _____

_____   _____

_____   _____

_____   _____

_____   _____

_____   _____

_____   _____

_____   _____

_____   _____

Calories Out:

Activity   Calories Burned

_____   _____

_____   _____

_____   _____

BMR: _____ Weight: _____ Date: _____

About the Author

Aaron Knipp has been stereotyped as 'the fat kid' for most of his life. By 19 he was over 320 pounds and thought there was nothing he could do. His whole life was defined by his weight and the limits that weight set for his future. Never would he imagine his newest title of personal trainer and fitness coach.

Aaron completely shattered his weight loss barriers and achieved his fitness goals, and now he wants to do the same for you.

It only took one moment, one experience, that pushed him to find the method that allowed him to lose 140 pounds in only two years. Now Aaron wants to help you achieve your weight loss and fitness goals and help kickstart your life on this road to health.

Aaron currently works as a personal trainer and fitness coach. If you want to book Aaron as a speaker for your event, please email him at aaron_knipp@aol.com.

Find Aaron Knipp online on these platforms:
Facebook: Aaron Knipp

Instagram: aaron_knipp
LinkedIn: Aaron Knipp
YouTube: https://www.youtube.com/channel/
UCrHuUHuw3FMh7g9hZZ56GMA

Made in the USA
Las Vegas, NV
10 June 2022

50074309R00105